Henry J Barber.

The Times

Alex a Rd,

Penzance

ATLAS OF NEUROPATHOLOGY

ATLAS OF NEUROPATHOLOGY

BY

WM. BLACKWOOD

M.B., F.R.C.S.E.

*Assistant Pathologist, the National Hospital, Queen Square, London ;
formerly Senior Lecturer in Neuropathology, University of Edinburgh,
Neuropathologist to the Scottish Mental Hospitals' Laboratory, the Royal
Infirmary, Edinburgh and Edinburgh Municipal and Emergency Medical
Services Hospitals*

T. C. DODDS

F.I.M.L.T., F.I.B.P., F.R.P.S.

*Laboratory Supervisor, Department of Pathology, University of Edinburgh ;
Lecturer to the Society of Radiographers (Fellowship Course) Scottish Branch*

AND

J. C. SOMMERVILLE

A.I.M.L.T.

*Senior Technician, the Department of Neuropathology, University of
Edinburgh and Scottish Mental Hospitals' Laboratory*

FOREWORD BY

PROFESSOR A. MURRAY DRENNAN

M.D., F.R.C.P.E., F.R.S.E.

Professor of Pathology, University of Edinburgh

EDINBURGH
E. & S. LIVINGSTONE LTD.
16-17 TEVIOT PLACE
1949

LRJAA

Printed in Great Britain by
McLagan & Cumming Ltd., Edinburgh

PREFACE

THIS atlas takes its origin from the demonstrations given over a period of many years to those studying neuropathology in the Laboratory of the Scottish Mental Hospitals and in the University of Edinburgh.

The material from which the illustrations have been obtained is a collection of slides and specimens built up successively by Professor J. H. Biggart, Dr. A. Colin P. Campbell and Dr. William Blackwood.

The purpose of the atlas is to try to present to clinicians or pathologists beginning the study of neuropathology the most important pathological conditions in a clear and simple way. It is intended for use in conjunction with the examination of actual specimens and preparations, with a systematic course of lectures or a text-book of neuropathology. For these reasons the scope of the book has been kept within certain limits. Neither in text nor in illustrations is it meant to be an advanced or comprehensive atlas. The reader may consider that there are many omissions, but some of these are deliberately made. In particular, we have tried not to overload the section on Tumours, restraining the natural impulse to include all their varieties and histological details. We have stressed instead the more important features of the displacements which may be produced by tumours. In the legends and the text we have tried to emphasize some of the main features and the basic principles of the pathological processes rather than include all the details.

This atlas could not have been made without the conscious or unconscious help of many people. In particular we should like to express our debt to Dr. A. C. P. Campbell, Professor Norman M. Dott, Professor A. Murray Drennan, Dr. J. G. Greenfield and the late Lieut.-Colonel W. F. Harvey, from whose personal teaching so much has been learnt ; to Professor J. H. Biggart who has kindly agreed to the arrangement of this atlas being similar to his " Pathology of the Nervous System " ; to the pathologists who have supplied us with some of the material illustrated, in particular to the late Lieut.-Colonel W. F. Harvey for the specimen of Schilder's disease and to Dr. Agnes Macgregor for the specimens of hepatolenticular degeneration and nuclear jaundice ; to the unrecorded gentleman who presented the anencephalic fœtus ; to those who have kindly allowed us to use their illustrations or utilize those of our own already published :— Percival, Drennan and Dodds' " Atlas of Histopathology of the Skin," 1947,

E. & S. Livingstone, Figs. 5 and 257. Low and Dodds' " Atlas of Bacteriology," 1948, E. & S. Livingstone, Figs. 56, 65 and 97. Le Gros Clark's " Tissues of the Body," 2nd edn. 1945, Oxford University Press, Fig. 3. Hamilton, Boyd and Mossman's " Human Embryology," 1945, W. Heffer, Figs. 234, 238, 239, 240, 241 and 242. Rowbotham's " Acute Injuries of the Head," 2nd edn., 1945, E. & S. Livingstone, Figs. 159 and 162. Thomson and Miles' " Manual of Surgery," 9th edn., 1939, Oxford University Press, Figs. 171, 191, 193, 194, 195 and 198. Miller and Davidson's " Practical Pathology including Morbid Anatomy and Post-Mortem Technique," 3rd edn., 1938, A. & C. Black, Fig. 36. *Post-Graduate Medical Journal* (Dr. Blackwood), Figs. 17, 42, 49, 64, 66 and 68. *Archives of Disease in Childhood* (Drs. J. G. Macleod and R. M. Macdonald), Figs. 153 and 154. *Journal of Pathology and Bacteriology* (Dr. A. C. P. Campbell and Professor J. H. Biggart), Figs. 123, 124, 125 and 126 ; (Dr. W. Blackwood), Figs. 259 and 260. *British Journal of Surgery* (Dr. W. Blackwood), Figs. 4, 6, 175, 176, 177, 183, 184 and 185. *Journal of Anatomy* (Dr. E. Gutmann and Professor J. Z. Young), Fig. 182. *The Lancet* (Dr. A. H. S. Holbourn), Fig. 163. *Edinburgh Medical Journal* (Dr. W. Blackwood), Figs. 178, 179 and 180. *British Journal of Ophthalmology* (Dr. W. Blackwood), Figs. 224 and 225. To Dr. L. G. Leitch, Mr R. W. Matthews and Mr C. Shepley for the drawing of Figs. 35, 57, 83, 143, 156 and 186, and for all the lettering on the illustrations ; to the clinical staff, both Honorary and Resident, of The Royal Infirmary, Edinburgh, The Royal Edinburgh Hospital for Nervous Diseases, Murray Royal, Perth, The Royal Hospital for Sick Children, Edinburgh, the Edinburgh Municipal and Emergency Medical Service Hospitals and the Deaconess Hospital, etc., for their co-operation and clinical notes, in particular the late Professor W. T. Ritchie for the case of hemichorea, Professor R. W. B. Ellis for the case of hepato-lenticular degeneration, Professor Sir David K. Henderson for the case of Pick's lobar atrophy, Huntington's chorea and senile dementia, Professor Norman M. Dott for nearly all the tumour and traumatic cases, as well as others ; to the many friends, including Dr. D. W. Liddell, Dr. L. Wolman and Dr. W. G. P. Mair who by suggestion or criticism have helped in the preparation of this atlas ; to the assistant technical staff, in particular Messrs. R. Russell, R. Allan, J. Paul and D. Wallace ; to Miss D. A. Lewendon for preparing the typescript ; to Miss J. B. Gardner for editing and proof reading ; and last but not least to the publishers for their courtesy and kindness and for rendering it possible to achieve a long cherished wish.

EDINBURGH AND LONDON THE AUTHORS.
November 1948.

CONTENTS

FOREWORD

To those entering upon the study of the special pathology of the nervous system it is necessary to have some visual conception of the pathological changes which are found. This is best attained by study of specimens, gross and microscopical, where a suitable collection is available. But where this is not convenient, or when it is desired to refresh the memory of these changes, recourse must be had to illustrations.

In the current textbooks of pathology and neuropathology there are, of course, excellent pictures of the main features of disease of the nervous system, but it is not possible to portray more than a limited number of these. Thus there emerges the need for some more extended collection such as appears in this atlas.

As the authors state, even this series does not profess to illustrate all pathological possibilities, but it sets out most of those likely to be met with in the ordinary course of neuropathology.

The great majority of the lesions shown are from the collection gathered by Dr. Blackwood and his predecessors while working as Neuropathologists in the Laboratory of the Scottish Mental Hospitals Scheme, now incorporated in the Neuropathological Department of the Department of Pathology in Edinburgh University. Some of the conditions shown have already been published, most of them appear here for the first time.

Unless the normal is known deviations from it cannot be appreciated. To help in this the authors begin with a brief account of the normal constituents and throughout there are inserted pictures of the normal alongside the pathological.

Mr Sommerville's beautiful technical work in the preparation of the original specimens has made possible the clear and convincing illustrations in monochrome or colour, which are the work of Mr Dodds.

The result is a combined effort of the pathologist, who identifies and selects the lesion, the technician who makes possible its detailed study and the artist who perpetuates it for all to see.

A.M.D.

ATLAS OF NEUROPATHOLOGY

SECTION I
NORMAL CYTOLOGY AND REACTIONS
TO DISEASE
INTRODUCTION

The following cells are found in the central nervous system. Each type of cell has a different function.

(1) **Nerve cells ;** the cell bodies are found only in grey matter. The complete unit, consisting of nerve cell with dendrites and axis cylinder, is called the neurone. It carries out the nervous functions of the brain and spinal cord.

(2) **Astrocytes ;** spider-like cells which are present throughout the central nervous system. They support the nervous tissue and repair damage.

(3) **Oligodendroglia ;** small cells found in both white and grey matter. They probably aid in the production and maintenance of the myelin sheaths.

(4) **Microglia ;** members of the reticulo-endothelial system, which normally occur throughout the central nervous system. They are stimulated to act as scavengers by the presence of dead tissue or abnormal substances (*e.g.*, senile plaques, Fig. 133).

No one stain shows all the cells, their nuclei, cytoplasm and processes at one time and selective stains are used in neuropathology to demonstrate certain structures only. Fig. 1 shows a portion of the cerebral cortex stained with thionin blue (Nissl's method).

NEURONE

In Fig. 1 a large nerve cell in the motor cortex is seen. Note the large central nucleus, poor in chromatin, with a single prominent nucleolus (this nucleolus is a diagnostic feature of a nerve cell). Note the large masses of dark staining Nissl substance, present throughout the cytoplasm except on the " axon hillock." Nissl substance is probably an iron-containing protein.

Neurofibrils (Fig. 2) run through the nerve cell, out along the dendrites and the axon. Formed of collections of large longitudinally orientated molecules of protein (Young, 1945), neurofibrils appear like thin wires when impregnated with silver. The axis cylinder or axon is composed of neurofibrils and of the non-fibrillar axoplasm which surrounds the neurofibrils (Figs. 2 and 3). The axon is covered, to a varying degree, in proportion to its calibre, by a fatty substance, myelin.

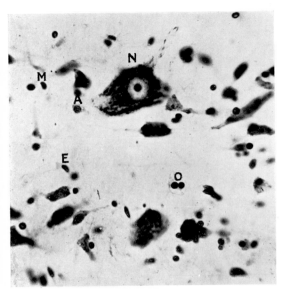

FIG. 1. *Normal pre-central cortex*, showing the cells stained by Nissl's method. Below (*N*) is a nerve cell, (*A*) an astrocyte, (*O*) two oligodendroglia, (*M*) a microglial nucleus and (*E*) a capillary endothelial cell nucleus. *Thionin blue* × 350.

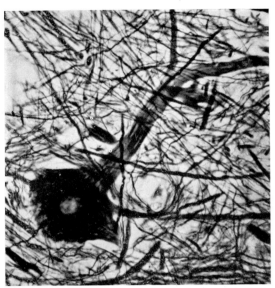

FIG. 2. *Anterior horn cell, spinal cord*, showing neurofibrils running through the cell cytoplasm. *Silver impregnation (Hortega)* × 350.

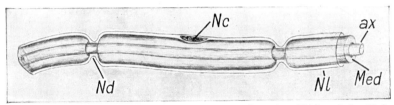

By courtesy of Professor Le Gros Clark.

FIG. 3. *Diagram illustrating schematically the essential structure of a medullated nerve fibre outside the brain or cord.* The axis cylinder or axon (*ax*) is enclosed in a medullary (*Med*) or myelin sheath and this again is surrounded by a fine sheath of neurilemma (*Nl*). Deep to the neurilemma lies a Schwann cell, only the nucleus of which (*Nc*) is shown. The medullary sheath is constricted between each Schwann cell at the nodes of Ranvier (*Nd*).

FIG. 4. *Peripheral nerve bundle in transverse section*, showing various sizes of myelinated nerve fibres. Each single fibre lies within its neurilemmal sheath, which is surrounded by a collagenous endoneurial sheath. Single fibres are grouped into bundles and surrounded by a thicker collagenous perineurial sheath (running obliquely top right to left centre in picture). In larger nerves, which consist of several bundles, the whole is surrounded by a collagenous epineurial sheath. *Weigert Pal.* × 280.

By courtesy of The British Journal of Surgery.

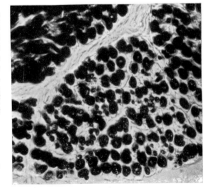

3

NEURONE

The axons of the peripheral nerves terminate in various types of endings which are specialized, either to send off impulses to the central nervous system (sensory endings) (Fig. 5), or to transmit nerve impulses from the central nervous system to other tissues (motor endings) (Fig. 6).

REACTION OF NEURONE TO DISEASE

The most important of the degenerative changes occurring in nerve cells is chromatolysis (lysis or disintegration of the chromophil substance or coloured part of the cytoplasm) (Fig. 7). Chromatolysis is a reversible reaction. If the nerve cell is injured to such a degree that it dies, that cell is never replaced by multiplication of other nerve cells or of germinal cells. Degenerative changes in nerve cells can readily be produced by post-mortem change or faulty fixation, so that changes such as those shown in Fig. 7 should always be interpreted with caution and search made for contributory definite evidence of cell reaction (*see* Figs. 90 and 91).

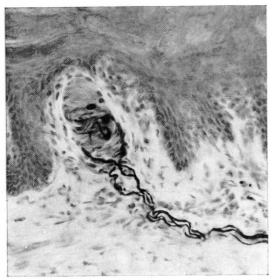

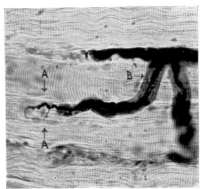

By courtesy of the The British Journal of Surgery.

FIG. 6. *Normal motor nerve ending in the hypothenar muscle.* The axon leaves the myelin sheath (*B*) just before the end plate (*A*) on the muscle fibre.

L.S. Axis cylinder stain × 265.

By courtesy of Professors Percival and Drennan and Mr Dodds.

FIG. 5. *Sensory nerve ending.* Meissner's corpuscle from the skin of the volar aspect of a finger. Mechanical deformation of the ovoid end corpuscle sends sensory impulses along the nerve fibres. *Silver impregnation (Weddell) and Carmine* × 260.

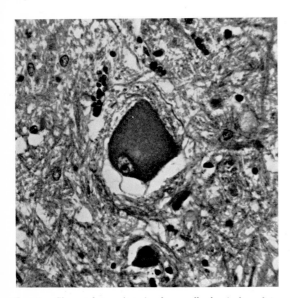

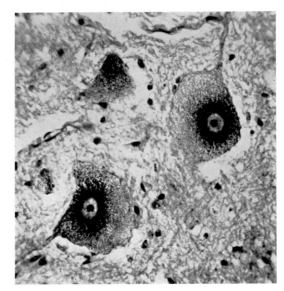

FIG. 7. *Chromatolysis.* Anterior horn cell of spinal cord in acute ascending paralysis. The cell is swollen and rounded, the Nissl substance is lysed except at the periphery and the nucleus is eccentric. Compare Fig. 1. (The clear space below the cell is an artefact due to shrinkage.)
Hæmalum and Eosin × 350.

FIG. 8. *Amaurotic family idiocy.* Anterior horn cells of spinal cord showing great distension and rounding off of the cell body due to the excess of lipoid. The Nissl substance lies centrally around the nucleus.
Thionin blue × 350.

ASTROCYTES

(star-shaped cells)

Two types of astrocytes occur : (1) **protoplasmic**, found only in the grey matter, and (2) **fibrillary**, found in both white and grey matter, though normally absent from layers II to V of the cortex and from the caudate nucleus, globus pallidus and putamen, except in the immediate neighbourhood of the ventricles and the larger vessels.

The processes of the protoplasmic astrocytes are shorter and they branch more frequently than those of the fibrillary astrocytes. Both types have at least one sucker foot attached to a capillary.

The function of the astrocytes is support under physiological conditions and repair or replacement (by fibrous astrocytes) under pathological conditions.

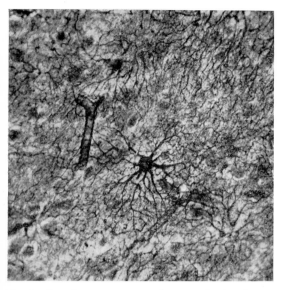

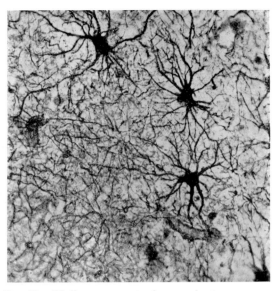

FIG. 9. *Protoplasmic astrocytes in the cortex* showing shorter, more frequently branching, finer processes, which give the cells a " mossy " appearance. They also have a " sucker foot " attached to a blood vessel. *Gold impregnation (Cajal)* × 350.

FIG. 10. *Fibrillary astrocytes in the cortex* showing numerous long processes, at least one of which is attached to a blood vessel. *Gold impregnation (Cajal)* × 350.

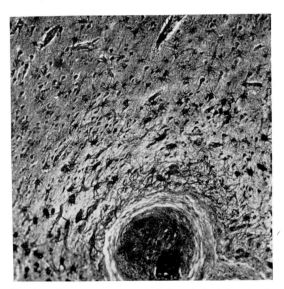

FIG. 11. *Reactive astrocytes.* A little embolic infarct in the cortex is seen. Note the increase in size (lower magnification than Figs. 9 and 10) and number of the astrocytes, which are forming a glial scar around the thrombosed vessel. *Gold impregnation (Cajal)* × 85.

OLIGODENDROGLIA

(oligo = few + dendron = branched + glia = glue)

These cells are found as (1) satellites of nerve cells in grey matter, (2) lying in long rows between the myelin sheaths in the white matter. They have no vascular foot plates.

Their processes are few and short. Their function appears to be that of aiding in the metabolism and life of myelin, for they appear with the myelin and disappear from areas of demyelination.

MICROGLIA

(micro = small + glia = glue)

Before metallic impregnations were employed, only the nuclei of these cells were visible. Since they have the smallest nuclei of the cells which " glue " together the nerve cells, they were called the microglia (small glue).

Normal microglial cells are difficult to stain except in fresh tissue. They have a small ovoid nucleus and branching mossy processes (Fig. 13).

Microglia are present throughout the brain and cord, especially in the grey matter. They are developed from mesoderm (neurones, astrocytes and oligodendroglia from ectoderm) and their function, analogous to that of other members of the reticulo-endothelial system, is essentially **histiocytic**, the removal of dead or foreign material. Normally they lie in a resting phase.

COMPARISON OF NORMAL ASTROCYTES, OLIGODENDROGLIA AND MICROGLIA			
FEATURE.	ASTROCYTE.	OLIGO-DENDROGLIA.	MICROGLIA.
NUCLEAR SIZE	relatively large	small	small.
SHAPE	oval	round	ovoid, kidney or rod shaped.
STAINING	hypochromatic	hyperchromatic	hyperchromatic.
CYTOPLASMIC PROCESSES	numerous, at least one attached to a blood vessel	few, no vascular process	few main processes which sub-divide repeatedly. No vascular process.
FUNCTION	support	associated with metabolism of myelin	phagocytic.
ORIGIN	ectoderm	ectoderm	mesoderm.

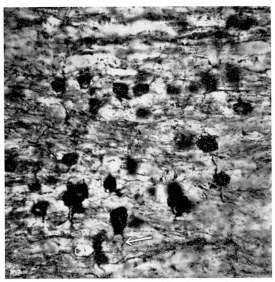

FIG. 12. *Oligodendroglia in the white matter*, lying in rows along the myelinated nerve fibres, showing a pale staining nucleus, dark staining cytoplasm and few short processes (arrow). This section is from a dog's brain. In human material they rapidly undergo post-mortem cytoplasmic swelling.

Silver impregnation (Hortega) × 350.

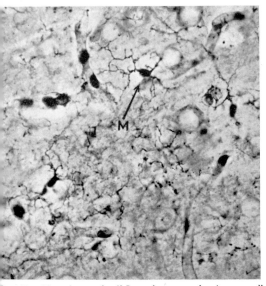

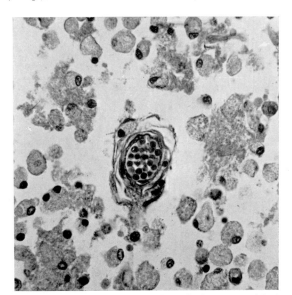

FIG. 13. *Normal microglia (M) in the cortex*, showing a small void nucleus and branching processes. This section is from a rabbit, in which the material is more easily obtained fresh than in man. The cell is similar in both.

Silver impregnation (Hortega) × 450.

FIG. 14. *Reactive microglia in an infarct.* In the presence of dead tissue these mobile cells show swelling of their processes (see Figs. 101 and 133). Eventually the cell becomes rounded off and full of phagocyted lipoid material which is carried off to the nearest perivascular space or thence into the vessel lumen. Such swollen cells, shown here, are called " compound granular corpuscles " or " gitter " cells. *Hæmalum and Eosin* × 350.

SECTION II

VASCULAR DISEASE

INTRODUCTION

The functions of the central nervous system are carried out by the nerve cells, their axons and dendrites. These require a good blood supply, and are rapidly damaged or killed by anoxæmia. When nerve cells die they are not replaced anatomically (*e.g.*, by division of existing nerve cells), but the lost function may be taken over by other neurones. Regeneration of axons in the peripheral nervous system may occur as long as the nerve cell is intact.

In spite of protective mechanisms, many factors may contribute to or cause anoxæmia of cerebral tissue. Such factors may be :—

(1) Abnormalities of the circulatory system outside the brain, *e.g.*, auriculo-ventricular heart block (giving rise to Adam Stokes syndrome), surgical shock.

(2) Abnormalities of the cerebral vessels, *e.g.*, of function as in hypertensives or following cerebral trauma : of structure such as atherosclerosis, syphilitic arteritis, arteriolosclerosis.

(3) Abnormalities of the blood in the vessels, *e.g.*, conditions associated with deficient oxygenation of the blood, thrombosis in arteries or veins, emboli, leukæmia, carboxyhæmoglobin in carbon monoxide poisoning.

ATHEROSCLEROSIS

The pathological process in the central nervous system is similar to that seen in the rest of the body. It commonly affects the larger vessels at the base of the brain, but may involve the smaller cortical or the perforating vessels. The occlusion is at first gradual, but may be accelerated by thrombosis upon the internal surface of the plaque.

Atherosclerosis of the rest of the body, especially of the coronary arteries, is often but not always accompanied by cerebral atherosclerosis, but cerebral atherosclerosis probably never occurs by itself.

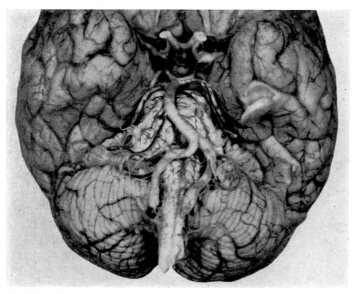

FIG. 15. *Atherosclerosis.* Base of the brain in a patient aged sixty-three years, with mental symptoms. Note diffuse and patchy flecking of the basal arteries with whitish (or yellowish) plaques of atheroma.

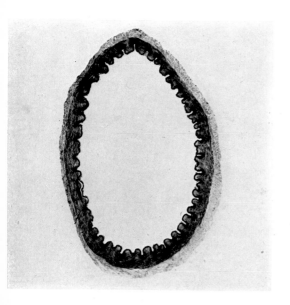

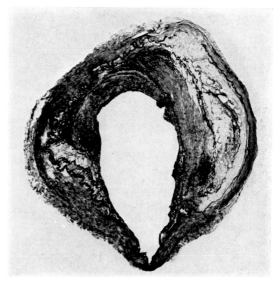

By courtesy of The Post-Graduate Medical Journal.

FIG. 16. *Normal basilar artery,* showing the crenated internal elastic lamina, the muscular media and the thin adventitial coat. *Trichrome stain (Masson)* × 30.

FIG. 17. *Atherosclerotic basilar artery,* showing eccentric sub-endothelial fibrous thickening with fatty change in the deeper part, eccentric splitting of the internal elastic lamina and fibrous replacement of medial muscle. *Trichrome stain (Masson)* × 30.

INFARCTION [cramming (with blood)]

Infarction, *i.e.*, death of tissue due to a reduction in blood flow below the necessary minimum, is due to obstruction of feeding or draining vessels, and may be caused by such conditions as thrombosis of an atherosclerotic artery; occlusion by syphilitic arteritis, or by embolism; or by venous thrombosis.

If the occlusion is gradual and the blood flow through the anastomotic channels is poor, as in atherosclerosis, the infarct tends to be pale.

If the occlusion be sudden and the blood flow through the anastomotic channels is good, either from absence of vascular disease or due to hypertension, the infarct will be red.

Initially an infarct tends to swell, later to shrink.

Whether an infarct due to arterial obstruction affects the grey matter or the white matter, or both, depends upon the size and anatomical distribution of the involved artery. If the vessel is very small, *e.g.*, an arteriole, then the lesion may be confined to either white or grey matter. If the vessel is larger, then both white and grey matter will be involved. If the involved vessel is a large one with a predominantly cortical distribution, *e.g.*, the middle cerebral artery in the stem of the lateral fissure, then the infarction will involve principally the cortical grey matter and a thin subjacent strip of white matter. Deep to these " U " fibres (Fig. 118) lies the " watershed " between superficial and deep blood supply.

The deep white matter is not supplied by separate arteries, but is supplied in common with the deep basal nuclear masses (caudate, lentiform, thalamus) by perforating vessels given off close to the circle of Willis. When any of these perforating vessels is blocked the infarct will involve both deep white matter and deep grey nuclei.

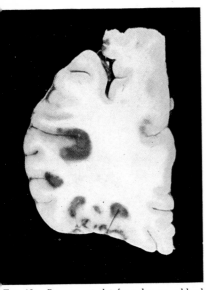

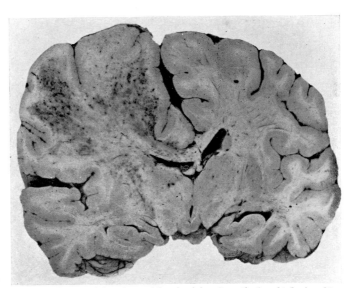

FIG. 18. *Recent cortical infarct* due to a bland embolus suddenly impacting, 30 hours before death, in the middle cerebral artery and causing infarction in its cortical distribution. The deep white matter is not visibly affected. Note the swollen and hæmorrhagic cortex.

FIG. 19. *Recent embolic infarct*, of five days' duration, affecting chiefly the white matter, in the zone of distribution of the central perforating branches of the middle cerebral artery. The infarct was very soft, greyish pink in colour, studded with petechial hæmorrhages. The vascular network is less dense in the white matter, so that the infarct is less red than in the cortex. There is swelling of the brain on the affected side (left in picture) due to œdema. This œdema may empty the blood vessels in some regions and give a " pale infarct."

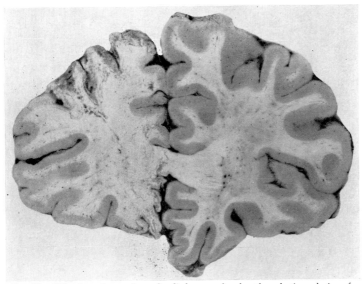

FIG. 20. *Old infarct*, in a patient who died ten weeks after thrombotic occlusion of a sclerotic anterior cerebral artery. There is an old hæmorrhagic infarct, chiefly cortical, on the left side of the picture, in the field of distribution of the anterior cerebral artery. Note how this side of the brain has shrunk (compare Fig. 19). Some gyri on the surface of the brain were depressed, wrinkled and pigmented yellow with hæmosiderin —" plaque jaune."

REACTION TO ACUTE ARTERIAL OCCLUSION

Beyond the vascular obstruction the initial reaction is one of vascular dilatation and slowing of the blood flow (pre-stasis or stasis). As a result of the slowing there is ischæmic damage to the capillary endothelium. Plasma leaks from the vessels, giving rise to œdema, and red blood corpuscles pass through their walls (diapedesis of red blood corpuscles) (Figs. 21 and 22). The diapedesis is most marked in the highly vascular grey matter (which in life is pink due to its rich vascularity, but goes grey after fixation). In the white matter the capillary meshwork and anastomoses are less dense (*see* Fig. 52), and the swelling due to œdema may squeeze the blood out of adjacent regions of the capillary bed (pale infarct) (Fig. 23).

The first cellular reaction is on the part of the blood-borne polymorphonuclear leucocytes (about 18 hours) (Fig. 24).

INFARCTION

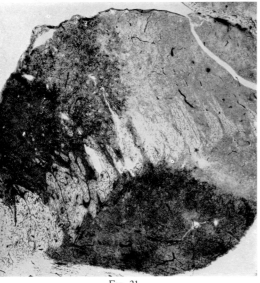

Fɪɢ. 21

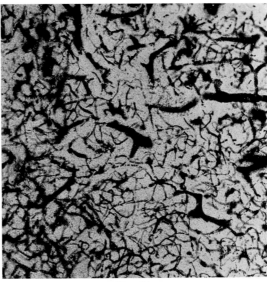

Fɪɢ. 22

ʒ. 21. *Recent (53 hour) embolic infarct of corpus striatum (caudate upper left, putamen lower right, internal capsule between). The* ʙbolism stopped the blood supply (recurrent artery of Heubner) to the structures in the lower left part of the illustration and there was ʙarction, which is less obvious in the white matter (internal capsule) than in the grey matter (caudate and putamen). (See Figs. 22 and) The normal vascular bed in the upper right part of the illustration acts as a control. *Thick frozen section. Pickworth preparation* × 4.

ʒ. 22. *Higher power view of portion of infarcted grey matter in Fig.* 21 showing the dilatation of the vascular bed. Fuzziness of the vessel ʇline indicates diapedesis of red blood corpuscles. *Pickworth preparation, in which the red blood corpuscles are selectively stained* × 50.

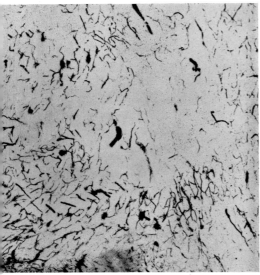

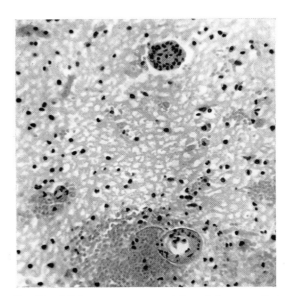

Fɪɢ. 24.

G. 23. *Moderately high power view of portion of infarcted* ʇernal capsule in Fig. 21, showing the normally less dense ʇpillary network and a pale region where the œdema is associated with poor filling of the vascular tree. *Pickworth preparation* × 15.

Fɪɢ. 24. *Cellular picture in a recent infarct of the grey matter,* showing the emigration of polymorphonuclear leucocytes into the œdematous dying parenchyma, from the vessels which are dilated and often leaking plasma and red blood corpuscles. *Hæmalum and Eosin* × 220.

15

REACTION TO ACUTE ARTERIAL OCCLUSION (CONTD.)

The microglia then react ; their processes swell and they engulf the necrotic tissue, becoming " compound granular cells " (about 3 days) (*see* Fig. 14). They remove the debris to the perivascular spaces and thence into the vascular lumen. Swelling of the astrocytes occurs in the less affected area round the infarct. The blood vessels become prominent due to swelling and possibly proliferation of their endothelial cells (Fig. 25). The cell debris is partially or wholly removed. Some phagocytes are always left behind, in and around the infarct. Phagocytes which contain hæmosiderin give a yellow tinge to the infarct.

Repair is carried out by the astrocytes, which lay down astrocytic (glial) fibres. Finally, the cystic space is surrounded by a wall of glial fibres and a decreased number of astrocytic nuclei (Figs. 26 and 27). Connective tissue (collagen), plays no significant part in the repair of an infarct of the central nervous system.

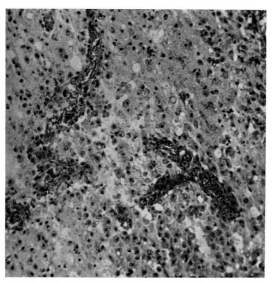

FIG. 25. *Infarct of grey matter of one week's duration* showing the prominence of the capillaries due to endothelial cell hyperplasia and the infiltration of the dying parenchyma by compound granular corpuscles (phagocytes swollen to rotundity by ingested cell debris). *Hæmalum and Eosin* × 110.

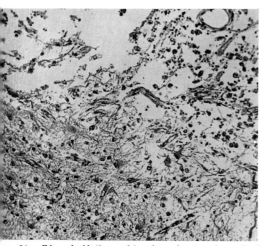

IG. 26. *Edge of old (3 months) infarct* showing the wall of trocytes and astrocytic fibres. Phagocytes, whose mobility has een impaired by their content of lipoid or hæmosiderin, are entangled in the glial fibres.
Mallory's phosphotungstic acid hæmatoxylin × 100.

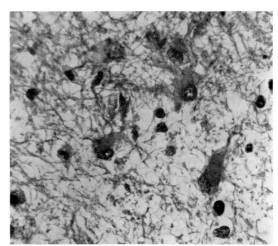

FIG. 27. *High power view of portion of Fig. 26,* showing the astrocytes and astrocytic fibres. As frequently happens in relatively ischæmic regions, many of the astrocytes have copious, hyaline-looking cytoplasm (gemästete or stuffed astrocytes).
Mallory's P.A.H. × 450.

THE EFFECTS OF VASCULAR DISEASE IN CERTAIN SITUATIONS

HEMIPLEGIA

One of the commoner manifestations of vascular disease in the brain is hemiplegia, due to interruption of the continuity of the motor pathway by hæmorrhage, thrombosis or embolism. This interruption most commonly occurs in the internal capsule.

The axis cylinders and myelin sheaths, being cut off from the nerve cells in the cortex, degenerate. As a result, the pyramid on the affected side is smaller and in the cord there is degeneration of the direct and crossed pyramidal tracts.

VASCULAR LESION IN THE PYRAMIDAL TRACT

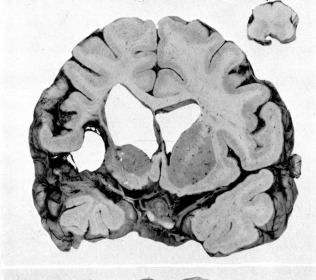

FIG. 28. *Anterior view of a coronal section of brain in a case of hemiplegia.* Many years ago occlusion of an atherosclerotic middle cerebral artery on the right side of the body (left side of picture) led to extensive infarction in its field of supply. Note the destruction of the central white matter and the internal capsule. Above the brain is a horizontal section of medulla (viewed from below) showing atrophy of the pyramid (arrow) on the same side as the lesion.

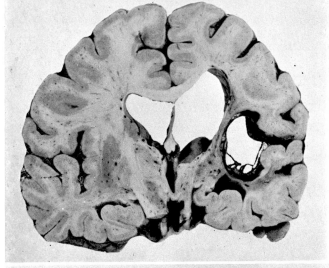

FIG. 29. *Posterior view of slice of brain seen in Fig.* 28 showing extensive destruction of internal capsule (also basal ganglia and insular cortex). Note the compensatory dilatation of the right lateral ventricle.

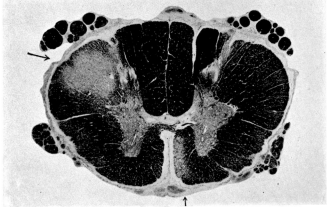

FIG. 30. *Hemiplegia.* Cervical cord showing degeneration in the crossed pyramidal tract, on the side opposite to the cerebral lesion and in the direct pyramidal tract, on the side of the cerebral lesion. The arrows point to these regions, where the normally dark staining myelin has degenerated. The section is mounted with the anterior portion downwards.
Myelin stain (Weigert Pal) × 7.

VASCULAR LESION IN THE CORNU AMMONIS

The hippocampal gyrus, in particular that part of it which is known as the cornu ammonis, is very susceptible to injury in ischæmic states of the brain. This finding may be connected with the anatomical features of its blood supply, for it is supplied by branches of a long fine artery, the anterior choroidal artery. The most easily damaged cells lie in the " vulnerable sector " (Fig. 32, *A* to *B*) of the pyramidal cell layer. Cell loss from this region does not give rise to any special clinical features. At one time it was thought that epilepsy arose from damage to the cornu ammonis, but it is more likely that the changes seen there are the result of the anoxæmia during epileptiform attacks rather than the cause. An identical picture of cell loss is commonly seen in pellagra and other forms of Vitamin B deficiency.

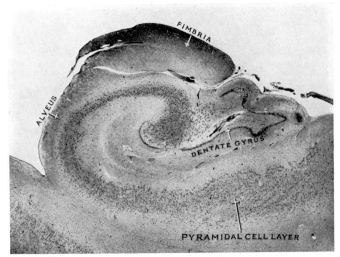

FIG. 31. *Normal cornu ammonis* (*ram's horn*), the part of the hippocampus which projects into the inferior horn of the lateral ventricle. Note the layer of large pyramidal cells which runs a curved course before ending in the embrace of the nerve cell layer of the dentate gyrus. *Thionin blue* × 9.

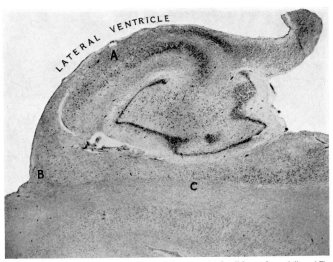

FIG. 32. *Cornu ammonis* showing loss of the pyramidal cell layer from (*A*) to (*C*). The portion (*A*) to (*B*), bordering the ventricle, is called Sommer's sector or the vulnerable sector. It is supplied by branches of a long fine artery, the anterior choroidal artery, and is very susceptible to anoxæmia. The specimen is from an elderly patient with cerebral atherosclerosis. Similar changes are found in epilepsy. *Thionin blue* × 10.

HEMIBALLISMUS OR HEMICHOREA

Clinical Note.—The patient was a woman aged 48 years, known to have had hypertension for many years. Twenty days before death there was a sudden onset of violent uncontrollable movements of the right arm and leg. At first these movements ceased during sleep, but later were continuous and uncontrolled by sedatives. She died from respiratory infection.

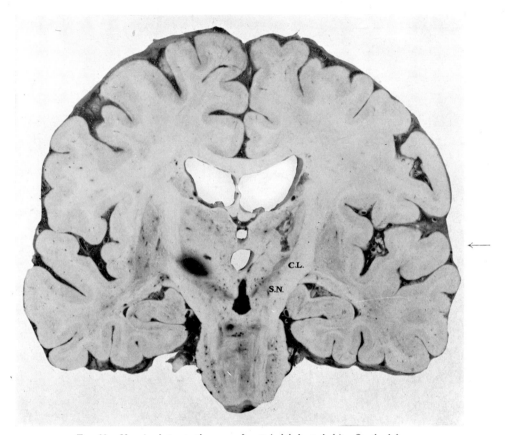

Fig. 33. *Vascular lesion in the corpus Luysii (subthalamic body).* On the left side the corpus Luysii is replaced by hæmorrhage. On the right side it (*C.L.*) is intact. The substantia nigra (*S.N.*) is not affected on either side. Note the old cystic infarct in the right thalamus and the atherosclerosis of the cortical arteries in the right insular region (2 cm. from brain margin at arrow). The clinical result of the lesion was hemiballismus or hemichorea.

POSTERIOR INFERIOR CEREBELLAR ARTERY
THROMBOSIS

Clinical Note.—The patient was a woman aged 58 years who, eight weeks before death, suffered from giddiness and later choking. Fourteen hours before death there was loss of sensation over the left side of the face (descending root of trigeminal nerve), weakness of the left facial muscles (facial nerve nucleus), paralysis of the left side of the palate and the left vocal cord (nucleus ambiguus), marked cerebellar signs in the left arm and the left leg with ataxia and dysdiadochokinesis (ventral spino-cerebellar tract and inferior cerebellar peduncle), loss of pain and temperature sense in the right arm and leg (lateral spinothalamic fibres), but no involvement of the pyramidal tracts.

Fig. 34 shows sections of her pons and medulla in which a darker infarcted region can be seen in the dorso-lateral aspect. The atheromatous basilar and vertebral arteries and the causative thrombus are seen below. Such patients may be ataxic (spino-cerebellar tracts involved) or may be vomiting, giddy and lying on the affected side (vestibular pathway involved). One side of the face may be paralysed (lower motor neurone lesion of the seventh nerve) and the patient feels as if cold or hot water were running down the face (partial involvement of descending root of fifth nerve with thermal dysæsthesia). The opposite side of the body shows loss of pain and temperature sensibility (*crossed* lateral spinothalamic pathway). Motor loss does not occur, since the pyramidal tracts are not involved.

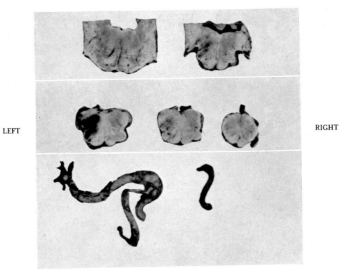

LEFT   RIGHT

FIG. 34. *Inferior aspect of slices of brainstem from lower pons to medulla in a case of thrombosis of the posterior inferior cerebellar artery.* This artery is a branch of the vertebral artery near its junction with its fellow to form the basilar artery. Below the slices of brainstem are the atheromatous basilar and vertebral arteries and the thrombus from the right vertebral artery. Note the hæmorrhagic infarct of the lower pons and upper medulla in the field of distribution of the artery, shown diagrammatically in Fig. 35.

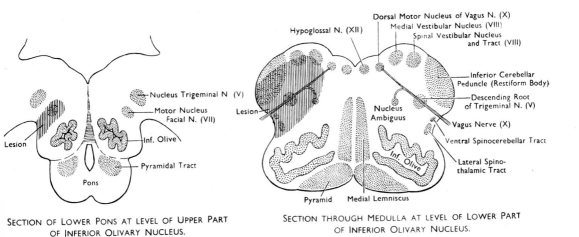

SECTION OF LOWER PONS AT LEVEL OF UPPER PART OF INFERIOR OLIVARY NUCLEUS.

SECTION THROUGH MEDULLA AT LEVEL OF LOWER PART OF INFERIOR OLIVARY NUCLEUS.

FIG. 35. *Diagram illustrating the lesion in thrombosis of the posterior inferior cerebellar artery.* The region usually infarcted is shaded on the left side.

HYPERTENSIVE CEREBRAL HÆMORRHAGE

The specimen (Fig. 36), is of a brain with the characteristic massive area of hæmorrhage, occurring in the bed of supply of the lenticulo-striate artery (once called " the artery of cerebral hæmorrhage ").

The theories as to the ætiology of massive cerebral hæmorrhage are many. The facts are that hypertension is always present and that the lesion is usually situated in the basal ganglia, pons or cerebellum.

Some theories are :—

(1) Rupture of Charcot's miliary aneurysms (actually adventitial hæmorrhages).

(2) Rupture of a diseased artery, the wall of which has degenerated from prolonged high blood pressure.

(3) Rupture of an artery whose supporting tissue has died from ischæmia (Globus and Strauss, 1927).

(4) Trauma to the arteriolar wall, caused by a wave of hypertension, producing a functional disturbance of the arterioles in the sense of Ricker. Focal arteriolar spasm occurs, with dilatation of the capillary bed beyond the spasm, with stasis of the blood flow, leakage of plasma and diapedesis of red blood corpuscles. Subsequent release of the spasm, in the presence of a good collateral blood supply, is followed by more extensive diapedesis and more vigorous and massive bleeding occurs (Grinker, 1943).

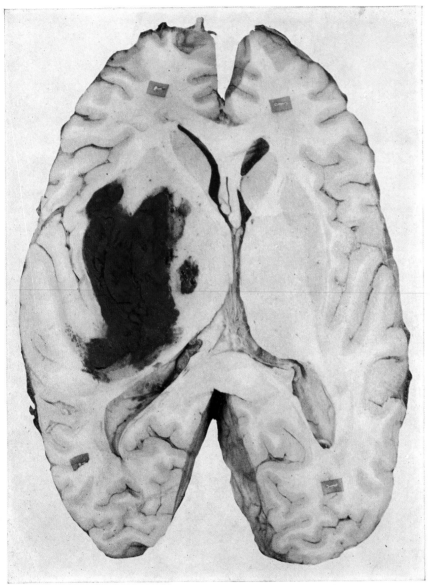

FIG. 36. *Horizontal section of brain* showing extensive hæmorrhage in the field of distribution of the lenticulostriate artery.

CONGENITAL ANEURYSM

These aneurysms usually occur on the arteries composing the circle of Willis and their larger branches. The aneurysm is usually found at a point of branching, but may occur at a site apparently remote from a branch. Such an aneurysm may be due :—

(1) To a congenital absence of the muscle of the medial coat at a point of branching.

In the normal development of the cerebral, mesenteric, coronary and probably all arteries, smaller arteries are not formed by budding from a larger one, but are formed each from a separate mass of mesoderm. Union subsequently occurs at the apparent point of branching. This union may be imperfect and the vessel wall at that point may be deficient in muscle and consist only of endothelium, elastic lamina and connective tissue. If the elastic lamina degenerates, the connective tissue will yield before the pressure of the blood and an aneurysm will develop (Forbus, 1930).

(2) To the weakening of the junction point between the anterior cerebral artery and the anterior communicating artery, not by any special mal-development of the vessel wall, but by the origin in the angle of junction, of several smaller branches (Drennan, 1921).

(3) To the imperfect absorption of an embryonic vessel which normally disappears as the vascular tree evolves (Dandy, 1944).

Microscopically the sac is composed of fibrous tissue. The elastica and muscularis cease at the neck of the sac. Such a sac is bound to yield before the relatively high blood pressure in the circle of Willis.

In older people, atherosclerosis, superimposed upon a congenital weakness, can contribute to the formation and rupture of such aneurysms.

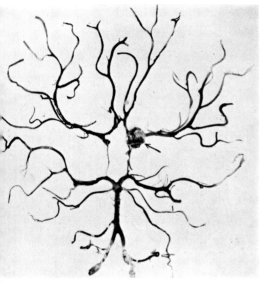

G. 37. *Dissected-out circle of Willis* showing (arrow) a congenital eurysm, of average size, arising at the origin of the ophthalmic tery from the internal carotid, in a woman aged thirty-nine years.

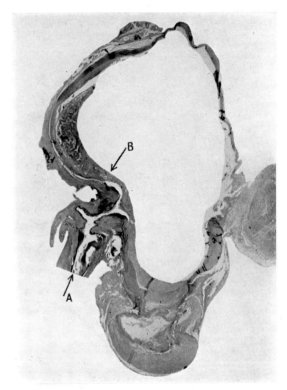

FIG. 38. *Congenital aneurysm* arising from an artery (*A*). The arterial wall opens out into the aneurysmal sac and the level of origin is indicated at (*B*). The sac has ruptured in a region opposite to the entrance point of the artery.
Elastic and Van Gieson stain × 11.

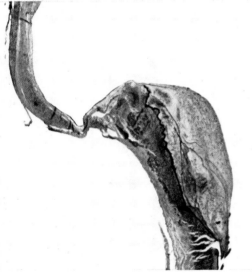

FIG. 39

FIG. 39. *Higher power view of region* (*B*) (*Fig.* 38) in another case. Below and to the right is the healthy arterial wall with black internal elastic membrane, purplish medial muscle and green adventitial collagen. About the centre of the picture there is a defect in the muscularis and elastic lamina, and beyond this lies the wall of the sac formed only of collagen. The purplish colour in the wall of the sac (top right) is due to artefact. Near the origin of the aneurysmal sac there is a plaque of intimal fibrosis. *Masson's trichrome stain* × 40.

CONGENITAL ANEURYSM

These aneurysms usually show themselves either by sudden massive subarachnoid hæmorrhage or by one or two small leakages and then sudden rupture. When these aneurysms rupture the blood may pass :—

(1) Into the cerebral tissue.

(2) Into the lateral ventricles.

(3) Into the basal subarachnoid space.

(4) Into the subdural space, if the aneurysm has leaked previously and so become adherent to the arachnoid. Then the arachnoid forms part of the wall of the sac and rupture occurs through it. This is relatively uncommon.

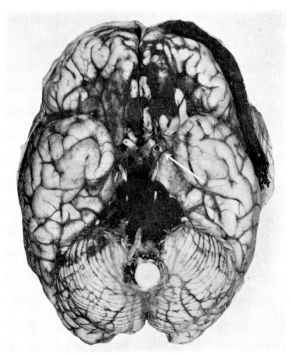

FIG. 40. *Inferior surface of brain* showing (arrow) a congenital aneurysm on the left middle cerebral artery which has ruptured both into the subarachnoid space (basal cisterns) and also into the subdural space. (Note blood clot on inner surface of dura top right of picture.)

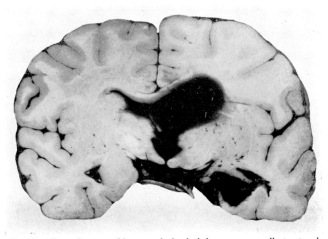

FIG. 41. *Coronal section of brain at the level of the corpora mamillaria viewed from in front.* A small aneurysm (not clearly seen) on the left middle cerebral artery has ruptured. The hæmorrhage is seen extending through the choroidal fissure into the inferior horn of the lateral ventricle and thus filling all the ventricular system.

INFECTIVE OR MYCOTIC ANEURYSM

Fig. 42 shows a section of brain in which a large hæmorrhage has occurred. This hæmorrhage is in relation to a thrombosed (middle cerebral) artery in a patient with subacute bacterial endocarditis in whom a septic embolus from the heart had impacted in the vessel. Infection of the wall had so weakened the vessel that a mycotic aneurysm was produced resulting in ultimate fatal rupture.

Such an aneurysm can occur only when the embolus is relatively large. Its commonest source is from left-sided endocarditis or from pulmonary infection. If the embolus is relatively small, then focal embolic encephalitis and its sequel, abscess formation, will develop.

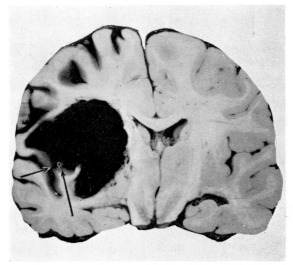

By courtesy of The Post-Graduate Medical Journal.

FIG. 42. *Coronal section of brain at the level of the substantia nigra, showing a massive cerebral hæmorrhage.* The arrows point to the middle cerebral artery whose wall had ruptured at this point due to secondary infection from an infected embolus.

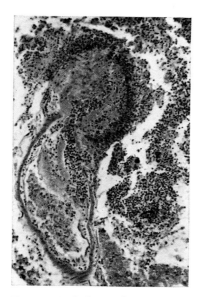

FIG. 43. *Cerebral artery showing a mycotic aneurysm.* The organisms in the infected embolus can be seen as a bluish haze at the periphery of the embolus. The arterial wall is weakened and bulging (upwards and to the right) and there has evidently been some leakage of blood. *Hæmalum and Eosin* × 80.

ARTERIOLOSCLEROSIS

Cerebral arteriolosclerosis consists of a fibrous thickening and narrowing of the small cortical arterioles, sometimes with "œdematous" splitting of the media. There may or may not be hyalinization of the fibrous tissue (as in the kidney in hypertension).

The disease process is a widespread one. Since the region of supply of an arteriole is small, the resultant brain lesions consist of multiple scattered *small* foci of anoxæmia (compare with atherosclerosis, Figs. 28 and 29).

Symptoms usually appear gradually, there is a tendency to temporary minor focal lesions and a relative rarity of hemiplegia. If a sufficient number of foci of cerebral atrophy are produced, there will be severe mental impairment and loss of intellectual ability going on to dementia.

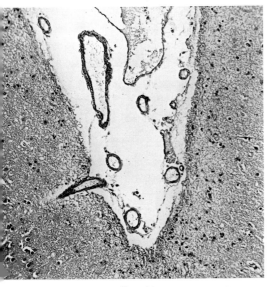
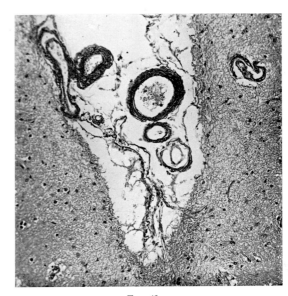

Fig. 44   Fig. 45

Fig. 44. *Normal cerebral arterioles* lying in a cortical sulcus.   The large vessel, incompletely shown top centre, is a vein.
Hæmalum and Eosin × 110.

Fig. 45. *Cerebral arterioles from a case of cerebral arteriolosclerosis.*   Note the fibrous thickening of the vessel walls.   The lowest of the three vessels in the centre shows the commonly found change of splitting of the media.   Note the arteriolar thickening within the cerebral tissue (top right) and the increase of subpial astrocytic nuclei and fibres.   *Hæmalum and Eosin* × 110.

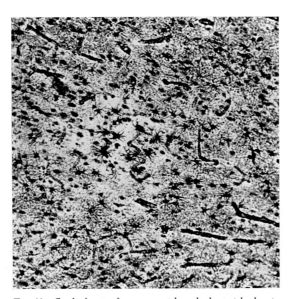

FIG. 46. *Cerebral cortex from a case with cerebral arteriolosclerosis,*
showing a focal pericapillary glial (astrocytic) scar in the centre of
the picture.   This is secondary to parenchymal damage.
Cajal's gold sublimate × 100.

35

FAT EMBOLISM

Clinical Note.—The patient was a woman, aged 67 years, who had been knocked down by a 'bus. She sustained, on one leg, a small wound which was sutured under general anæsthesia. The same night she became unconscious and remained so until her death four days later.

Fig. 47 shows a portion of her brain with the white matter studded with petechial hæmorrhages.

Microscopically there were numerous fat emboli present in the capillaries of both white and grey matter. In the white matter, where the capillary anastomosis is less dense, there were numerous ring hæmorrhages around capillaries, the walls of which were often necrotic.

Though commonly following bony trauma or manipulation of fractures, fat embolism can, as here, occur without obvious fracture, but with trauma to adipose tissue. The action of the fat is chiefly that of simple blockage. It is possible, however, that some of the fat is hydrolysed by lipases and that the fatty acids and resulting soaps are intensely irritating, causing damage to the capillary endothelium and subsequent necrosis and hæmorrhage.

FAT EMBOLISM

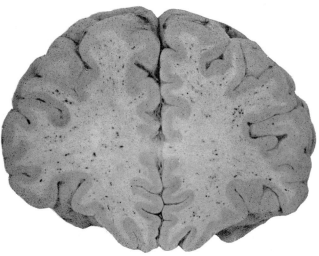

FIG. 47. *Coronal section of frontal lobes, in a case of fat embolism,* showing the multiple petechial hæmorrhages, predominantly in the white matter.

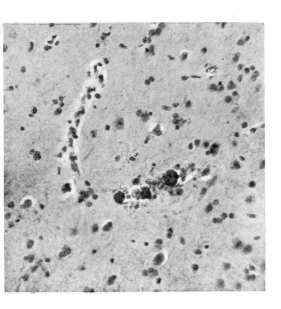

FIG. 48. *Portion of cerebral cortex in a case of fat embolism,* showing fat globules in a cortical capillary. *Sharlach R. hæmalum* × 200.

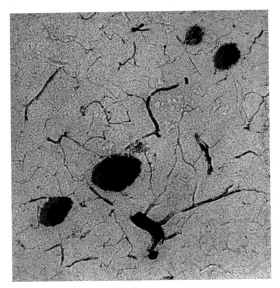

By courtesy of The Post-Graduate Medical Journal.

FIG. 49. *Cerebral white matter, case of fat embolism,* showing the capillary hæmorrhages. *Thick frozen section, Pickworth preparation* × 30.

37

VENOUS THROMBOSIS (EARLY)

Figs. 50 and 51 show aseptic thrombosis of the superior sagittal sinus in a child with vomiting and diarrhœa. Note the hæmorrhagic discolouration and crumbling consistence of the right occipital region. Infective venous sinus thrombosis commonly follows suppuration in the nasal air sinuses or middle ear and mastoid air sinus, in the scalp or the bones of the calvarium. It can also follow parturition, especially when there has been pelvic infection. In these cases it is probable that emboli reach the cranium by retrograde venous emboli passing up the paravertebral and intravertebral venous systems.

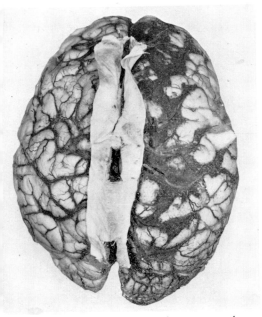

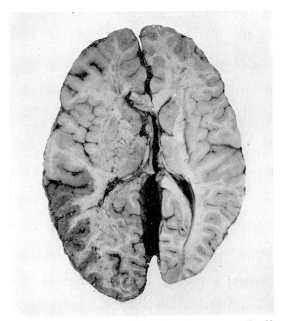

FIG. 50. *View of brain and dura from above in a case of recent septic venous sinus thrombosis.* The superior sagittal venous sinus has a window cut in it to show the thrombosis. The entering veins on the right side are distended and thrombosed, and there is much subarachnoid hæmorrhage around them.

FIG. 51. *Horizontal section of brain from the same case as Fig.* 50, *viewed from below,* showing the venous infarction of the cortex, especially in the occipital (lower) region. Note the swelling of the affected hemisphere.

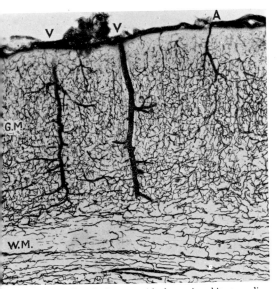

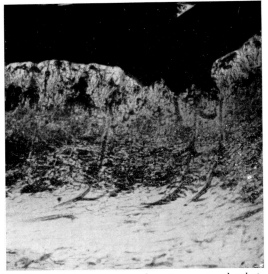

FIG. 52. *Normal cerebral cortex* with the angioarchitecture displayed by staining the red blood corpuscles within the vessels. *V* = vein, *A* = artery, *G.M.* = grey matter, *W.M.* = white matter. The veins branch more frequently and the branches come off more at right angles than the arteries. *Pickworth preparation* × 20.

FIG. 53. *Cerebral cortex in a case of recent venous sinus thrombosis.* The veins are dilated and leaking blood, much of which has found its way, in the perivascular spaces, up to the surface. The subarachnoid space (top of picture) is full of blood. *Pickworth preparation* × 15.

SECTION III
ORGANISMAL INFECTION

PYOGENIC INTRACRANIAL INFECTION
ACUTE PURULENT LEPTOMENINGITIS. BRAIN ABSCESS. SEPTIC THROMBOSIS OF DURAL VENOUS SINUSES

Pyogenic infection of the intracranial structure may arise :—

(1) **From a neighbouring focus**, *e.g.*, in the ear, nasal cavity, nasal accessory air cavities, or the scalp, face, etc. From such a focus the infection may reach the intracranial structures by—

A. DIRECT EXTENSION THROUGH BONE

   (*a*) Traumatic fracture.
   (*b*) Osteomyelitis.

The infection spreading through the bone may give rise to extra-dural abscess, venous sinus thrombosis, subdural abscess, generalized acute purulent leptomeningitis or brain abscess.

B. EXTENSION BY THE VENOUS SYSTEM

A small vein at the primary focus is thrombosed, and infected clot spreads continuously or by emboli to a dural venous sinus. From here septic thrombosis may spread along the tributory veins (pial and intracerebral), causing acute purulent leptomeningitis or brain abscess.

C. EXTENSION ALONG PREFORMED ANATOMICAL PATHWAYS

   (*a*) The perineural lymphatics of the olfactory nerve.
   (*b*) The pial sheath of the optic nerve.
   (*c*) The aqueduct of the cochlea.

Infection by these pathways gives rise to acute purulent leptomeningitis.

(2) **From a distant focus** being blood-borne to the brain or the lepto-meninges. The commonest primary focus is in the lung, from which the infection travels chiefly by the arterial blood stream. Pyogenic intracranial infection may also follow pelvic infection, without inter-mediary pulmonary infection, in which case it is probable that the route is via the paravertebral and intravertebral venous systems.

ACUTE PURULENT LEPTOMENINGITIS (MENINGOCOCCAL)

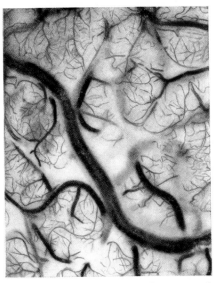

FIG. 54. *Cerebral cortex in a case of meningococcal leptomeningitis.* The surface is very congested and the creamy coloured purulent exudate is most abundant in the regions where the subarachnoid space is large, *e.g.*, along the sulci (as shown), in the basal cisterns and around the cauda equina. A large vein runs across the field.

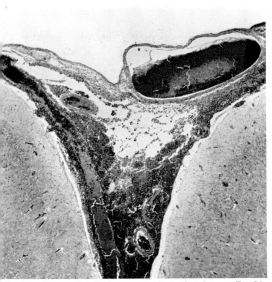

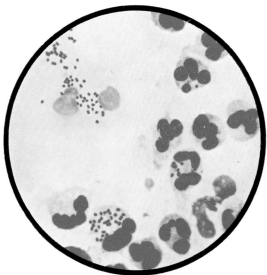

By courtesy of Dr Low and Mr Dodds.

FIG. 55. *Section of cerebral cortex, similar to that shown in Fig. 54,* in a case of acute purulent leptomeningitis, showing the cellular exudate in the subarachnoid space of a cerebral sulcus. Note the dilated blood vessels (vein top right, artery lower centre). *Hæmalum and Eosin* × 10.

FIG. 56. *Exudate in the subarachnoid space in a case of acute purulent leptomeningitis (meningococcal),* showing the numerous cells (polymorphonuclear leucocytes), many of which contain gram negative meningococci. Many organisms are also present extracellularly. *Gram's stain* × 1000.

41

BRAIN ABSCESS

Brain abscesses are usually multiple if the infection is blood-borne from a distant focus (when the route is most commonly by the arterial system) : single if coming from neighbouring structures (when the route is most frequently retrograde by the venous system). An abscess will occur only if the virulence of the organism is relatively low, or if the resistance of the host is relatively high. The lesion commences as a small focus of acute encephalitis, which enlarges. As it enlarges it becomes gradually circum-scribed by reactive fibrosis and (astrocytic) gliosis, so that a capsule is eventually formed. This capsule is not equally thick all the way round. It is usually thinner on the side nearest a free surface, *e.g.*, cortex, or a ventricle. Should further enlargement of the abscess occur, it does so in the direction of the free surface and may even rupture into the subarachnoid space or into the ventricle.

Fig. 59 illustrates a section of the brain of a man who received a per-forating wound of the stomach from a shell fragment. After operation he developed a subphrenic abscess, which cleared up, and a left-sided empyema which, in spite of surgical drainage, became chronic. The lower lobe of the lung collapsed and bronchiectasis developed in it. From here blood-borne organisms passed to the brain and set up an acute abscess. First he had a focal epileptiform attack, then gradually right hemiparesis, dysarthria and dysphasia developed. He was operated upon and one abscess drained. Thereafter fresh abscesses developed by retrograde septic venous thrombosis, and each was drained. Fig. 59 shows these older encapsulated abscesses lying towards the cortical surface. Finally a large, more acute, more central abscess developed, with ragged congested walls. This produced widespread œdema and a shift of midline structures to the right and led ultimately to death (from secondary upper brainstem hæmorrhage (*see* p. 140).

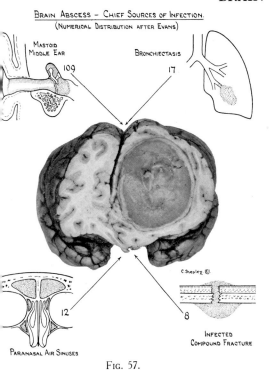

BRAIN ABSCESS – CHIEF SOURCES OF INFECTION.
(NUMERICAL DISTRIBUTION AFTER EVANS)

MASTOID
MIDDLE EAR
109

BRONCHIECTASIS
17

C. Shepley (E).

12

8

INFECTED
COMPOUND FRACTURE

PARANASAL AIR SINUSES

FIG. 57.

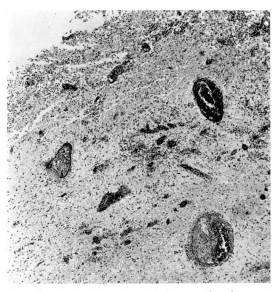

FIG. 58. *Cerebral tissue from the advancing edge of an acute abscess.* The picture is one of an acute encephalitis with spread chiefly by retrograde septic venous thrombosis. One of the involved veins is seen in the lower right corner of the picture. *Hæmalum and Eosin* × 45.

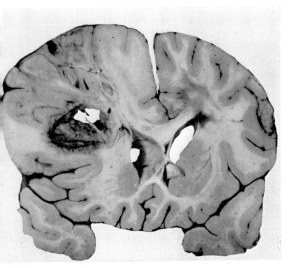

FIG. 59. *Coronal section of brain with multiple abscesses.* The older, better encapsulated abscesses lie towards the cortex. A large recent abscess lies near the ventricle. Note the surrounding œdema with displacement of midline structures.

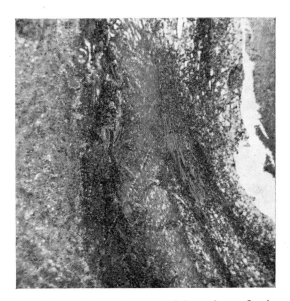

FIG. 60. *Wall of a well encapsulated brain abscess.* On the right is the pus (probably now sterile) within the abscess : then comes the collagenous wall (green) and, on the left, the outer layer of astrocytic gliosis (reddish), separated from the collagen by inflammatory cells. *Masson's trichrome stain* × 50.

43

TUBERCULOUS INFECTION

Cerebral tuberculosis is always secondary to tuberculosis elsewhere (*e.g.*, pulmonary or intestinal tuberculosis).

Whilst large solitary tuberculomata are rare, many cases of generalized tuberculous leptomeningitis can be traced to the presence of one or more tubercles, of relatively small size, in the substance of the central nervous system or in the leptomeninges, which eventually rupture and flood the leptomeninges with large numbers of tubercle bacilli (Rich *et al.*, 1933).

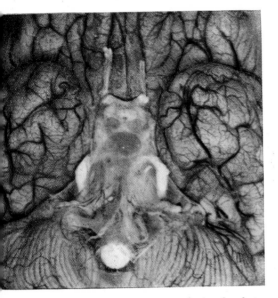

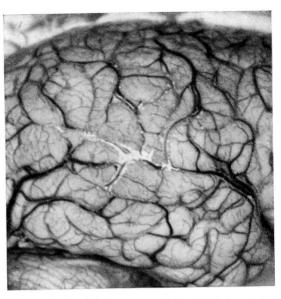

FIG. 61. *Inferior aspect of brain in a case of tuberculous lepto-meningitis* showing the tough greyish exudate in the basal (especially interpeduncular) cisterns. Scattered minute grey tubercles can be seen with difficulty (arrow) in the leptomeninges around the obvious exudate.

FIG. 62. *Surface of the brain in a case of tuberculous leptomeningitis.* The aggregation of small tubercles in the centre of the picture was found to overlie a small tuberculoma in the depth of the sulcus.

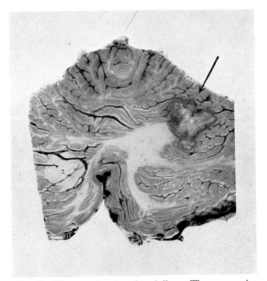

FIG. 63. *Horizontal section of cerebellum.* The arrow points to a tuberculoma, showing the irregularly shaped outline of the capsule and the caseous centre. Such a tuberculoma may grow in size, may calcify, or may rupture into the subarachnoid space or into a ventricle.

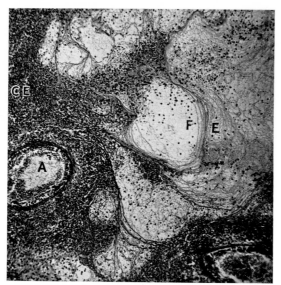

By courtesy of The Post-Graduate Medical Journal.

FIG. 64. *Exudate in the subarachnoid space in a case of tuberculous leptomeningitis,* showing the abundance of fibrin (*FE*), the copious cellular exudate (*CE*), predominantly mononuclear, and the arterial involvement (*A*). (See Fig 66.)
Hæmalum and Eosin × 60.

FIG. 65. *Cerebro-spinal fluid, from a case of tuberculous leptomeningitis,* after standing for some time in a test tube. Note the " spider web " clot composed of fibrin. Compare with the abundant fibrin seen in Fig. 64.

By courtesy of Dr Low and Mr Dodds.

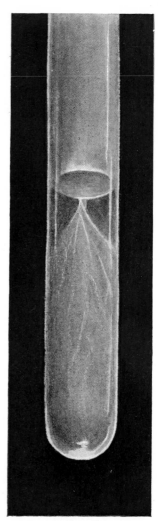

FIG. 65

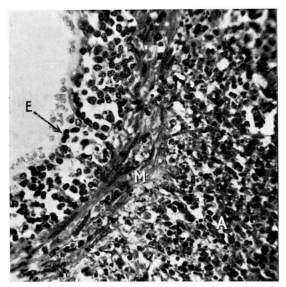

By courtesy of The Post-Graduate Medical Journal.

FIG. 66. *Higher power view of an artery in tuberculous lepto-meningitis* showing the subendothelial (*E*), medial (*M*), and adventitial (*A*) infiltration by lymphocytes and histiocytes. Necrosis of the arterial wall and thrombosis in the lumen are common sequelæ, with ischæmic damage to the underlying brain.
Hæmalum and Eosin × 350.

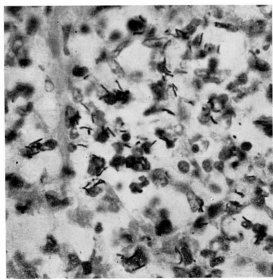

FIG. 67. *Subarachnoid space in a case of tuberculous lepto-meningitis* showing very numerous tubercle bacilli, mostly extracellular. *Ziehl Neelsen stain* × 950.

SYPHILIS

There are three ways in which syphilis may affect the central nervous system :—

(1) Meningeal (*acts by exudate*).

(2) Vascular (*acts by ischæmia*).

(3) Parenchymatous (*causes dègeneration*).

They may be found separately or together.

Meningovascular syphilis. The tempo and severity of the process can vary from a mild chronic inflammatory process to a more rapid, gummatous process.

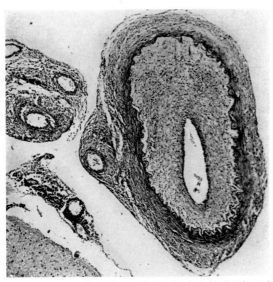

By courtesy of The Post-Graduate Medical Journal.

FIG. 68. *Cerebral artery in meningovascular syphilis* showing marked concentric intimal fibrosis. The internal elastic lamina and the media are damaged, but less conspicuously. There is an infiltration of all regions by lymphocytes and plasma cells. *Hæmalum and Eosin* × 40.

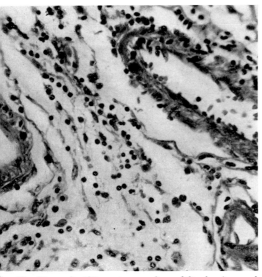

IG. 69. *Pia-arachnoid in meningovascular syphilis*, showing much xudate of lymphocytic, plasma cell and histiocytic type filling he meshes of the pia-arachnoid. Increased fibrous tissue hickens the meshwork. *Hæmalum and Eosin* × 350.

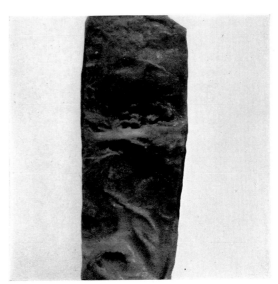

FIG. 70. *Deep surface of dura in gummatous pacchymeningitis.* There is fibrous and gummatous (necrotic fibrous tissue) thickening of the dura.

PARENCHYMATOUS SYPHILIS (G.P.I.)

This affects the brain and occurs 5-25 years after the primary infection. There is destruction of nerve cells which is so widespread as to lead to dementia. The neuronal destruction results in cerebral atrophy. Cellular exudate fills the subarachnoid space. The products of nerve cell destruction are taken up by the microglia and there is widespread reparative astrocytic gliosis. This gliosis occurs not only in the cortex and white matter, but also in the sub-ependymal region of the ventricles, where it gives rise to " granular ependymitis " (Figs. 81 and 82).

Fig. 72 is from a case of G.P.I. (" General paralysis of those already insane "). The leptomeninges are thickened and opaque because of the cellular exudate in the subarachnoid space. From loss of parenchyma the convolutions are atrophied and the sulci wider than usual. The leptomeninges have been stripped from one cerebral hemisphere.

Microscopically (Fig. 74) the cortex shows disturbance of cell architecture. The normal laminar pattern of the cortex is lost. Some nerve cells have been destroyed ; others are dying. Many of the survivors show a disturbance of their normal orientation, the apical dendrite pointing sideways instead of straight towards the surface. The cell population is not decreased for microglia are numerous (Fig. 77), and there is astrocytic proliferation (Figs. 80 and 81). Note the perivascular " cuffing " [plasma cells, lymphocytes and iron-containing histiocytes in the perivascular space (Fig. 75)]. Similar cellular infiltration is seen in the leptomeninges.

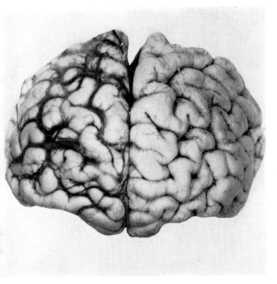

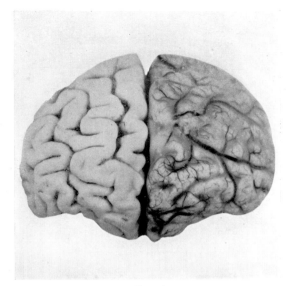

FIG. 71   FIG. 72

Fig. 71. *Normal frontal lobes*   On the right side of the picture the leptomeninges have been removed.

Fig. 72. *Frontal lobes in G.P.I.*   On the left side of the picture the leptomeninges have been removed to show the gyral atrophy and the resulting increased width of the sulci.   On the right side the cellular exudate in the sub-arachnoid space gives a cloudy appearance.

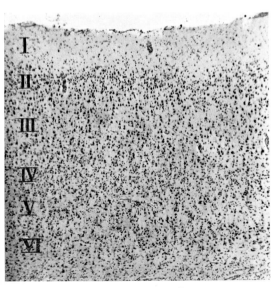

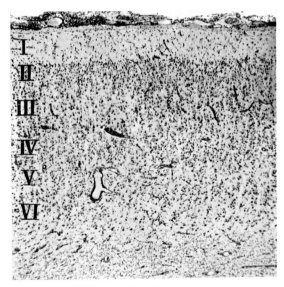

FIG. 73   FIG. 74

Fig. 73. *Normal frontal cortex.* The figures indicate the cell layers.   *Thionin* × 30.

Fig. 74. *Frontal cortex in G.P.I.* There is loss of nerve cells and increase of glial cells, so that the nuclear population is not decreased, but the cell layers are less distinct.   Note the cellular exudate around the vessels (lower left) and in the subarachnoid space (top of picture).   *Thionin* × 30.

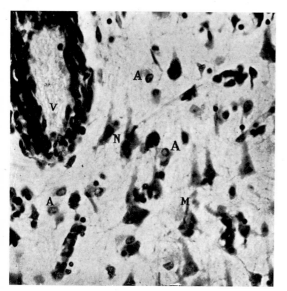

Fig. 75. *Cerebral cortex in G.P.I.*, showing degenerating nerve cells (either side of *N*), an increased number of astrocytes (*A*), the elongated nuclei of microglia (rod cell, below *M*) and the mononuclear exudate (lymphocytes, plasma cells and iron-containing histiocytes) in the Virchow-Robin space around a vessel (*V*). *Thionin* × 350.

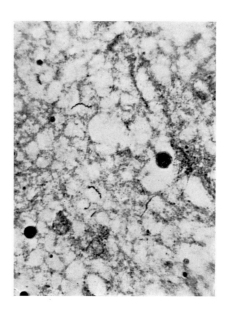

Fig. 76. *Cerebral cortex in G.P.I.* stained to show the spirochæte, *Treponema pallidum.* *Jahnel's silver nitrate impregnation* × 900.

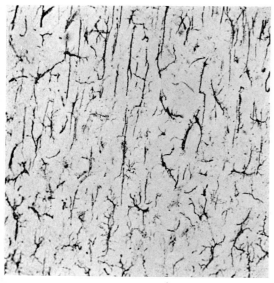

Fig. 77. *Cerebral cortex in G.P.I.* stained to show microglia. They are found to be increased in number and have an elongated shape (rod cells). Here both the cell nucleus and processes are stained. *Hortega's silver impregnation* × 110.

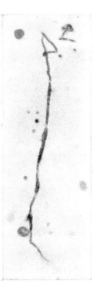

Fig. 78. *Rod cell in G.P.I.* showing the iron (blue staining) in the cell cytoplasm. Nuclei stain red. *Prussian blue reaction and carmine* × 700.

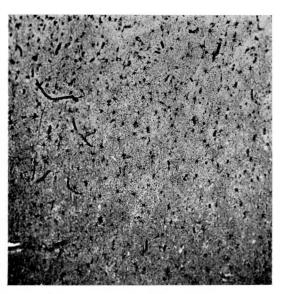

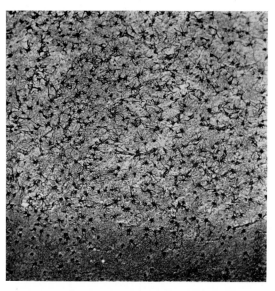

FIG. 79. *Normal cerebral cortex* stained to show astrocytes. The lowest part of the picture represents white matter.
Cajal's gold sublimate × 60.

FIG. 80. *Cerebral cortex in G.P.I.* stained to show astrocytes, showing the marked gliosis. The lowest part of the picture represents white matter. *Cajal's gold sublimate* × 60.

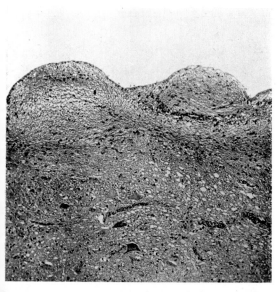

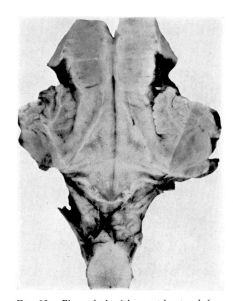

FIG. 81. *Floor of the 4th ventricle in G.P.I.* showing the characteristic " granular ependymitis." There are focal astrocytic glial nodules which often break through the overlying ependyma. *Hæmalum and Eosin* × 90.

FIG. 82. *Floor of the 4th ventricle viewed from above, in a case of G.P.I.,* showing the minute raised nodules which are indicative of " granular ependymitis."

4B

PARENCHYMATOUS SYPHILIS—TABES DORSALIS
(*wasting of the dorsal or posterior columns*)

Tabes dorsalis is not to be considered as primarily a disease of the posterior columns, but a disease starting at some point on the central prolongation of the ganglion cells of the (sensory) posterior nerve root.

Whatever the mechanism, the result is that the posterior roots degenerate at some point between the ganglion and the cord. The anterior (motor) roots are not involved.

The sensory fibres do not degenerate as a whole, but are thought to degenerate in groups which are relatively localized anatomically and physiologically. **Normally** the entering sensory fibres separate into three groups.

(1) SHORT FIBRES carrying impulses related to pain, the sensory side of the reflex arc, temperature (and some touch). These fibres synapse in the same segment in the posterior or, probably in the case of the reflex arc, in the anterior horn of the same side. (In Fig. 83 the reflex arc is shown with an intermediate neurone.)

(2) MEDIUM LENGTH FIBRES carrying impulses destined for the cerebellum and related to posture. These fibres [which are not collaterals of the long fibres, group (3), for the long fibres do not give off collaterals (Cajal)], synapse within a few segments in the cells of Clarke's column in the thoracic cord, or in the lateral cuneate nucleus (of Clarke-Monakow) in the lower medulla. On their way to the synapse, these fibres run for a short distance in the part of the posterior white column which lies in a middle zone between its anterior and posterior borders and is called the external bandalette of Pierret (which corresponds to the *middle root zone* of Flechsig, a name given by him to a zone in the cord which is not myelinated in a foetus of 24 cms. but is myelinated in one of 28 cms.). For the situation of the external bandalette *see* Fig. 84.

(3) LONG FIBRES carrying impulses related to muscle and joint sense, vibration and touch. These fibres run up in the posterior white columns to synapse in the nucleus gracilis and the nucleus cuneatus. Near their commencement they lie in a lenticular mass on the posterior and postero-medial aspect of the cord, but as they ascend they are displaced medially (*see* Fig. 84). They lie in the *posterior root zone* of Flechsig.

In **tabes dorsalis** these three fibre groups are progressively affected in approximately the same order as enumerated above. The involvement leads to impairment or loss of function, but the anatomical degeneration goes only as far as the first synapse. The cord degeneration, in myelin preparations, in a *very early case*, will therefore probably (for it is very difficult to demonstrate) be only in the short fibres which go at once to the posterior or anterior horns. In an *early case* the degeneration affects the short and medium length fibres and the conspicuous degeneration will be in the external bandalette of Pierret (*see* Fig. 84). In a *well developed case* the degeneration will also be in the long ascending fibres of the fasciculus gracilis and the fasciculus cuneatus (of Goll and Burdach), *see* Fig. 86.

The clinical changes correspond. The first sensory loss is that of pain. Whilst the pain fibres are degenerating they may give rise to spontaneous discharge phenomena, interpreted by the brain as pain (lightning pains). With complete degeneration there is analgesia. Next the afferent side of the reflex arcs disappears, first the deep reflexes (loss of knee jerks); then the sensory fibres which subserve muscle tone and position sense (producing hypotonia and ataxia, hence the clinical name " locomotor ataxia "). Later still the degeneration of the fibres carrying touch impulses leads to stocking anaesthesia.

TABES DORSALIS

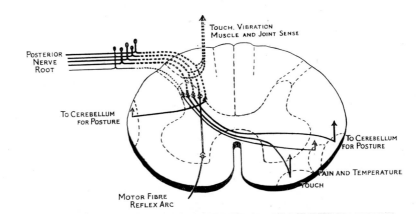

FIG. 83. *Diagram (after Ranson) of the main sensory inflow into the cord.* In a well-developed case of tabes dorsalis the lesion causes interference with the function of all entering fibres but the myelin degeneration (interrupted lines) proceeds only to the next synapse.

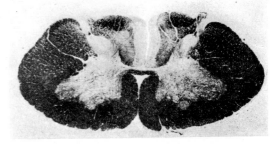

FIG. 84. *Cervical cord in a case of tabes dorsalis which was advanced in the lumbar region, less severe in the cervical region,* showing (1) the marked degeneration (region of pallor), in the fasciculus gracilis, of fibres which entered the cord in the lumbar region ; (2) degeneration, in the middle zone of the fasciculus cuneatus, of the external bandalette, composed of locally entering medium length fibres going to the external cuneate nucleus ; (3) preservation (black), in the posterior zone of the fasciculus cuneatus, of the locally entering long fibres going to the nucleus cuneatus. *Weigert Pal stain* × 5.

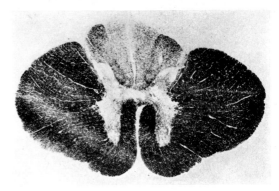

FIG. 85. *Thoracic cord in tabes dorsalis,* showing healthy myelin black, degenerate myelin pale. The oblique pallor in the antero-lateral column is artefact. *Weigert Pal stain* × 5.

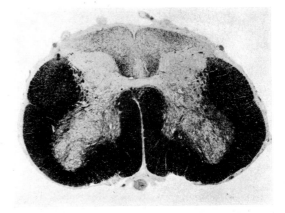

FIG. 86. *Lumbar cord in a well-marked case of tabes dorsalis,* showing the marked wasting of the posterior white columns due to the degeneration of all the entering fibres. *Weigert Pal stain* × 5.

GLIOSIS IN THE POSTERIOR COLUMNS OF THE CORD

In tabes dorsalis there is well-marked demyelination of the posterior white columns of the cord. There are two other conditions in which there is well-marked demyelination in the posterior white columns; these are subacute combined degeneration of the cord and Friedreich's ataxia. In both these diseases, however, the lateral columns are involved. The reaction on the part of the astrocytes in the three diseases is, however, quite different, so that sections stained for *astrocytic fibres* show three different pictures (Figs. 87, 88 and 89).

In **tabes dorsalis** there is dense gliosis of an isomorphic type, *i.e.*, the glial fibres are laid down parallel to the degenerated myelin.

In an **untreated case of subacute combined degeneration of the cord** there is very little gliosis. In a case treated with liver extract there is some gliosis, but it is not as dense as in tabes. In subacute combined degeneration of the cord large clear spaces, so characteristic of the condition, are seen.

In **Friedreich's ataxia** the gliosis is again dense, but it is in the form of characteristic whirlwind or " tourbillon " formations in the vicinity of small vessels.

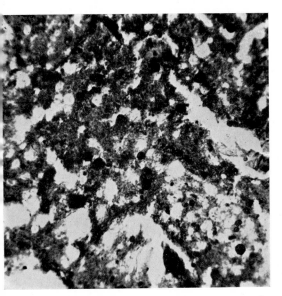

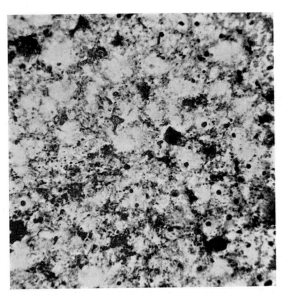

FIG. 87. *Posterior white columns in* **tabes dorsalis,** seen in horizontal section, after staining for astrocytic fibres. The very numerous astrocytic fibres of the isomorphic gliosis are seen in cross section. *Anderson's Victoria blue* × 200.

FIG. 88. *Posterior white columns in* **subacute combined degeneration,** seen in horizontal section, after staining for astrocytic fibres. There is very little gliosis in this condition. *Anderson's Victoria blue* × 200.

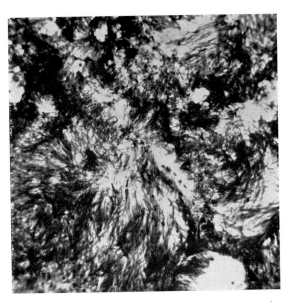

FIG. 89. *Posterior white columns in* **Friedreich's ataxia** seen in horizontal section, after staining for astrocytic fibres. There is very marked gliosis with a whirlwind (tourbillon) pattern around small blood vessels. *Anderson's Victoria blue* × 200.

VIRUS INFECTIONS

INTRODUCTION

The neurotropic viruses are usually obligatory neuronal parasites. They are thought to enter the peripheral extension of a nerve cell (*e.g.*, autonomic nerves of alimentary tract in acute anterior poliomyelitis) and then work their way within nerve cell substance, towards or into the central nervous system. The function of the nerve cells is impaired and the cell is often killed. Inclusion bodies may be present in the cell (rabies). In acute lesions there is necrosis of the nerve cells with a widespread microglial and mesodermal inflammatory reaction.

The different virus infections can seldom be distinguished from each other by the cellular response which they produce, but they do however tend to affect different levels and cell groups of the central nervous system, *e.g.*, acute anterior poliomyelitis attacks chiefly the grey matter of the anterior horns of the cord : encephalitis lethargica attacks chiefly the grey matter of the upper brain stem (3rd nerve nuclei and substantia nigra) and hypothalamus.

ACUTE ANTERIOR POLIOMYELITIS

(grey cord inflammation)

The virus is thought to pass from the alimentary tract, sometimes from the tonsils, to the brainstem and/or spinal cord via the automatic nerve fibres. At first the process may involve both anterior and posterior grey horns, the lesion in the posterior horns giving rise to pain on pressure of the muscles. But the main lesion is in the anterior horn cells giving rise to paralysis of the muscles. The nerve cells are not all equally involved. Some are destroyed (permanent paralysis) : some recover (transient paralysis) : some are not damaged. The illustrations show stages in the disease. In the early days the cell reaction is chiefly by polymorphonuclear leucocytes and microglia. The polymorphonuclear leucocytes are soon replaced by lymphocytes. These inflammatory cells pass up the perivascular spaces into the general cerebro-spinal fluid pathway and may appear in the fluid taken by lumbar puncture.

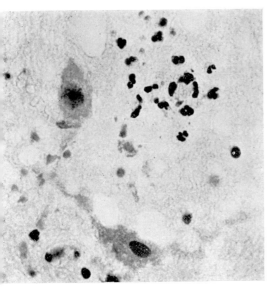

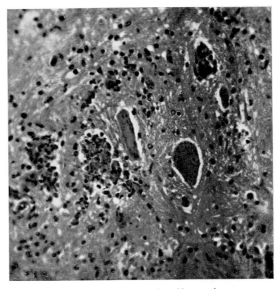

FIG. 90. *Anterior horn in an early (36-hour) case of acute anterior poliomyelitis*, showing two nerve cells undergoing chromatolysis and the remains of a third nerve cell, which is dead and surrounded by polymorphonuclear leucocytes.

Hæmalum and Eosin × 550.

FIG. 91. *Anterior horn in a four-day-old case of acute anterior poliomyelitis*. Some nerve cells are relatively healthy ; some are dying, their remains being smothered in a mass of polymorphonuclear leucocytes, lymphocytes and microglia. Lymphocytes surround a vessel in the top right-hand corner of the picture.

Hæmalum and Eosin × 200.

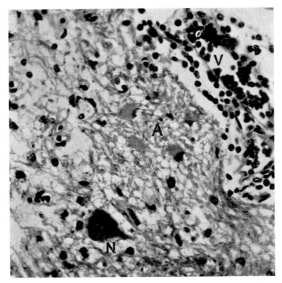

FIG. 92. *Anterior horn from a later case of acute anterior poliomyelitis*, showing that astrocytic scarring (*A*) has replaced the dead nerve cells. Another nerve cell (*N*) is recovering. There is still marked perivascular lymphocytic cuffing around a vein (*V*).

Hæmalum and Eosin × 350.

61

ENCEPHALITIS LETHARGICA
(*Sleepy Sickness*)

Although it has not yet been proved to be due to a virus, the histological picture is similar to that of infection by a neurotropic virus, with primary neuronal destruction and a secondary inflammatory reaction, which takes the form of perivascular cuffing by lymphocytes and an infiltration of the tissue by lymphocytes and microglia. If the disease takes the more common chronic form the histological picture is less active looking.

The process is usually most marked in the basal ganglia and brainstem, but it may be present in the cerebral cortex and gives rise to mental impairment (in the acute stage this gives the clinical picture of an acute toxic psychosis). In the chronic form of the disease, mental impairment and Parkinsonism are two of the clinical forms. Whatever the form of the disease, the substantia nigra is almost invariably damaged so that the process can be most easily followed at this level (Figs. 93 to 96).

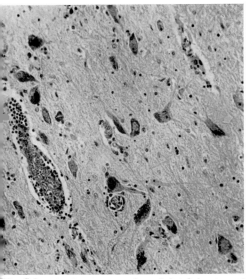

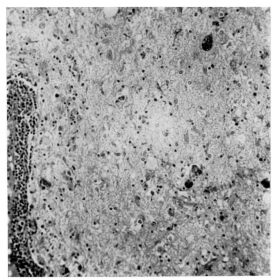

93. *Substantia nigra in a case of encephalitis lethargica with days' history.* A few of the pigmented nerve cells are dying ad ; their melanin is in phagocytes. There is perivascular lymphocytic cuffing in the Virchow-Robin space. *Hæmalum and Eosin* × 150.

FIG. 94. *Substantia nigra in a case of encephalitis lethargica dying after three weeks' history.* Many nerve cells are destroyed. There is cellular infiltration of the parenchyma and perivascular space (left side of picture) by lymphocytes and histiocytes. *Hæmalum and Eosin* × 150.

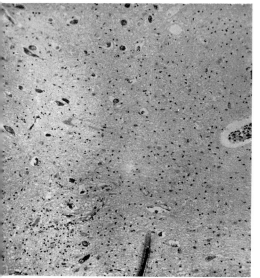

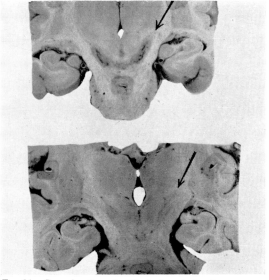

95. *Substantia nigra in a case of encephalitis lethargica of months' duration.* The tempo of the process has been slower. re is some general loss of nerve cells with focal accentuation a microglial response visible in the lower left corner of the ure. Note the lack of marked gliosis, since there has been little myelin destruction. *Hæmalum and Eosin* × 95.

FIG. 96. *Coronal sections of midbrain through the substantia nigra (arrow).* The upper specimen is from a healthy brain, the lower from a case of post-encephalitic Parkinsonism, where the bleaching of the substantia nigra is an indication of the severe damage to its nerve cells.

RABIES

The virus enters the body through the bite of a rabid dog, or, in Trinidad, the bite of a vampire bat. The histological picture is similar to but less severe than that seen in acute anterior poliomyelitis, but the localization is different, being commonly in the brainstem and basal ganglia. Negri bodies (Fig. 97) are not always demonstrable in human cases, being common in animals, especially in the hippocampal region. There may be small focal collections of microglial cells (glial " stars " or Babes' nodes) in the region of damaged nerve cells.

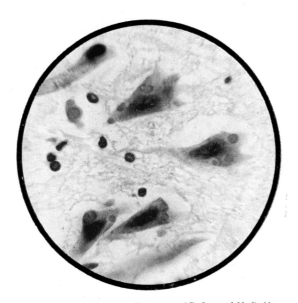

By courtesy of Dr Low and Mr Dodds.

FIG. 97. *Section of the hippocampus of a rabid dog,* showing the numerous rounded acidophilic intra-cytoplasmic inclusion bodies (Negri bodies).
Hæmalum and Eosin × 1,000.

SECTION IV

DEMYELINATING DISEASES OF UNKNOWN AETIOLOGY

POST-VACCINIAL ENCEPHALOMYELITIS

About the tenth day following vaccination, especially when done for the first time in an older child or an adult, there may develop an acute encephalomyelitis, involving both white and grey matter, characterized histologically by a widespread peri-venular demyelination. A similar encephalomyelitis may follow smallpox, chickenpox, measles and anti-rabic inoculation. The possibilities are that—

(1) It is due to the virus of the primary infection.

(2) It is not due directly to the virus of the primary preceding infection but to another virus, " which is either stimulated to activity or is directed against the nervous system by the exanthem." (Greenfield, 1929).

Clinical Note (Figs. 98-101).—The patient, a male aged $15\frac{1}{2}$ years, was admitted in coma, sixteen days after first vaccination, with a six days' history of progressive malaise and stupor. On examination there were signs of meningitis and a flaccid palsy of the lower limbs with retention of urine. *At autopsy* the brain, on section, showed only congestion, but *microscopically* the changes illustrated were seen in the brain and the cord.

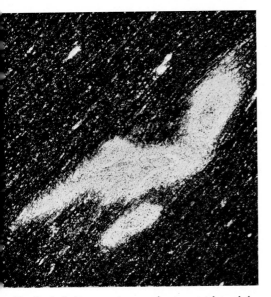

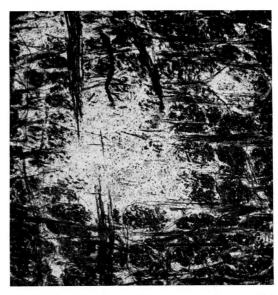

G. 98. *Cerebral white matter in a case of post-vaccinial encephalo-elitis, showing the perivenular demyelination. The venules can be seen faintly in the centres of the pale areas.*
Myelin stain × 20.

FIG. 99. *Reticular substance of pons in a case of post-vaccinial encephalomyelitis, showing the perivenular demyelination and the cellular infiltration of the demyelinated region.*
Myelin stain × 60.

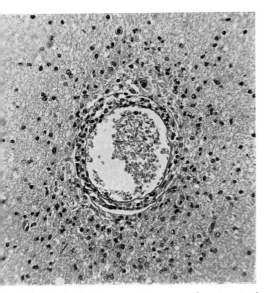

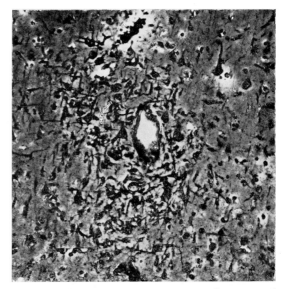

G. 100. *Cerebral white matter in a case of post-vaccinial cephalomyelitis, showing the cellular infiltration, both in the irchow-Robin space (" cuffing ") and in the parenchyma round the venule. Parenchymal infiltration is not " cuffing."*
Hæmalum and Eosin × 200.

FIG. 101. *Cerebral white matter in a case of post-vaccinial encephalomyelitis, stained to show microglia. This demonstrates that the greater part of the reaction to the destroyed myelin is by microglia, whose swollen processes stain darkly.*
Silver impregnation × 140.

DISSEMINATED SCLEROSIS

Clinical Note.—The patient was a man aged 28 years, who was admitted with a three years' history of difficulty in walking and shakiness of the hands. Examination showed intention tremor, nystagmus, increase of knee and ankle jerks and absence of abdominal reflexes. He was re-admitted six years later comatose, moribund, with loss of palatal and bladder reflexes.

Specimen (Fig. 102).—This was a well-marked case of disseminated sclerosis. Well-defined grey plaques of demyelination were present in brain and cord. They can be seen in the brain at the angles of the lateral ventricles (a common site), and in the white matter.

Microscopically (Figs. 105, 106 and 107) the majority of the plaques were old, though a few appeared to be more recent. In the old ones there was complete demyelination, a minor degree of axis cylinder loss and well-marked reparative gliosis of isomorphic type (*i.e.*, astrocytic fibres running in the line of the destroyed myelin).

Comment.—This is a disease of the myelin of undiscovered ætiology. Putman and Alexander (1939) think that the plaques of disseminated sclerosis are the result of occlusion of veins in the white matter by a thrombus composed of fibrin, platelets and leucocytes. Other views of the pathogenesis are—

    (1) Upset of enzyme system in relation to myelin (Hurst, 1941).
    (2) Virus infection.
    (3) Toxin of unknown origin.
    (4) Presence of a lipolytic enzyme in the blood plasma.
    (5) Spirochætal infection.

The multiplicity of theories is evidence of the lack of real knowledge.

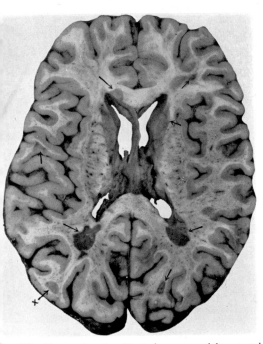

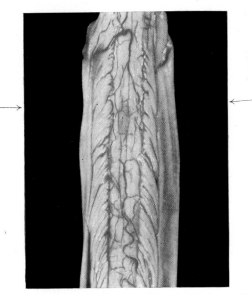

FIG. 103. *Cervical cord from a case of disseminated sclerosis.* The arrows point to the greyish surface discolouration which indicates an underlying "*plaque.*"

IG. 102. *Horizontal section of brain from a case of disseminated clerosis.* The arrows point to the numerous well-defined "plaques." They are greyish in colour due to the loss of myelin nd to the replacement gliosis. Note how they tend to lie either ound the ventricles or close to the cortex, involving both white nd grey matter, *cf.* Schilder's disease (Fig. 108). The lowest ight-hand plaque appears to surround a vein. It is more recent nd had a granular yellowish appearance when freshly cut. The rrow marked "X" points, not to a "plaque," but to the cut depths of a gyrus.

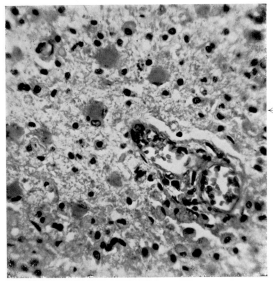

IG. 104. *Cerebral white matter in an early "plaque" of diseminated sclerosis,* showing the numerous plump astrocytes (one inucleated (arrow)), fat phagocytes (in the lower right-hand orner of the picture) and the mononuclear cells (lymphocytes and histiocytes) in the perivascular space.
Hæmalum and Eosin × 300.

FIG. 104

DISSEMINATED SCLEROSIS (contd.)

These three illustrations show the characteristic picture of an old cerebral plaque. The centre of the picture is approximately the edge of the plaque.

Fig. 105.—Stained by Spielmeyer's method for myelin sheaths. Note the clear-cut edge where the myelin sheaths end.

Fig. 106.—Neighbour section to preceding illustration stained by Hortega's silver method for axis cylinders. This shows that, although some axis cylinders are destroyed, many of them persist. This accounts for the slight degree of ascending and descending tract degeneration seen in cord sections compared to the number of plaques.

The process destroys the myelin and the associated œdema produces an additional physiological blockage of nervous impulses in the surrounding tissue—this is the attack. As the œdema subsides nerve impulse transmission can occur again—stage of remission.

Fig. 107.—Neighbour section to preceding one, stained Anderson's method for astrocytic fibres. Note that the gliosis is " isomorphic," i.e., the fibrils run in strands parallel to the destroyed myelin and not in an irregular meshwork.

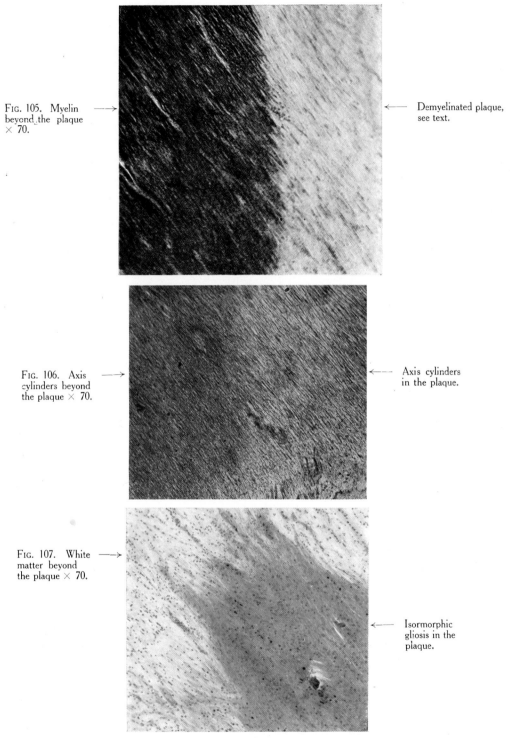

FIG. 105. Myelin beyond the plaque × 70.

Demyelinated plaque, see text.

FIG. 106. Axis cylinders beyond the plaque × 70.

Axis cylinders in the plaque.

FIG. 107. White matter beyond the plaque × 70.

Isormorphic gliosis in the plaque.

SCHILDER'S ENCEPHALITIS
(ENCEPHALITIS PERIAXIALIS DIFFUSA)

This is one type of diffuse cerebral sclerosis and is sometimes called progressive degenerative subcortical encephalopathy. It consists of a widespread degenerative process which usually starts in both occipital lobes and spreads forward through the cerebral white matter. A noticeable feature is the sparing of the subcortical arcuate (or " U ") fibres.

Clinically the disease is commonest in the first ten years of life, but has occurred up to the sixties. It manifests itself in cerebral blindness, mental impairment and progressive spastic paralysis.

Fig. 108 shows the change found in the left hemisphere (the right was similar). There is a granular appearance and softening of the white matter of much of the occipital lobe. The softenings are well demarcated. The " U " fibres are noticeably spared.

Microscopically.—The lesion had a sharply defined edge. Within it there were only fragmentary portions of myelin sheaths. The axis cylinders had suffered relatively little damage, compared to the myelin sheaths. The destroyed myelin was present in the form of lipoid in the vast numbers of compound granular cells which were present. The astrocytes were not increased in number (hence the softness of the region), but they had swollen cytoplasm (gemästete or " stuffed " astrocytes, *cf*. Fig. 27).

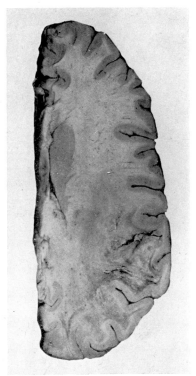

Specimen by courtesy of Col. Harvey.

FIG. 108. *Horizontal section of one cerebral hemisphere from a case of Schilder's disease.* The occipital pole is at the lower part of the picture. Note the granular soft appearance of the white matter of much of the occipital lobe, with the characteristic sparing of the white matter just deep to the cortex (subsulcine, arcuate or " U " fibres). The damaged white matter is not always soft ; it may be firm and greyish due to gliosis and loss of myelin.

SECTION V

INTOXICATIONS AND DEFICIENCIES

PERIPHERAL NEURITIS

Neuritis may be **interstitial** when the primary lesion is an inflammatory process in the connective tissue elements of the nerve, such as may affect a nerve passing through an abscess ; or **parenchymatous** if the primary lesion is a degeneration of the neural elements. In this second type the term " neuritis " is perhaps a misleading word, for the process is really a degeneration rather than an inflammation. It is a non-specific reaction which may follow vitamin deficiency (B1), the toxic influence of bacterial (diphtheria) or chemical (lead, arsenic) poisons : or in localized form from trauma (pressure of tumour, laceration, Saturday night paralysis of the radial nerve or chilling).

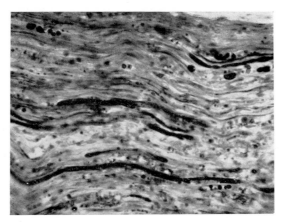

FIG. 109. *Longitudinal section of external popliteal nerve from a case of alcoholic polyneuritis* Note the severe loss of myelin. The dark globules are the unabsorbed remains of degenerating myelin. Compare with Fig 110.
Myelin stain × 180.

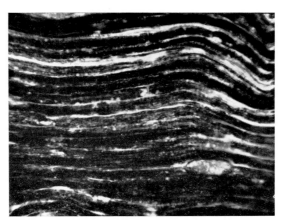

FIG. 110. *Longitudinal section of normal external popliteal nerve stained for myelin.* The swelling on a nerve fibre in the lower right-hand part of the picture is presumably a post-mortem artefact.
Myelin stain × 180.

ACUTE HÆMORRHAGIC ENCEPHALITIS (ARSENICAL)

Clinical Note.—The patient, a sailor, aged 33 years, contracted syphilis in 1941, for which he had four intravenous injections in Spain. No more treatment until 1944 when he was admitted with a positive blood Wassermann's reaction, but no clinical symptoms. His cerebrospinal fluid showed a strongly positive Wassermann's reaction and contained 50 cells per c.mm. (lymphocytes). The globulin was slightly increased and Lange's gold curve was 0012100000. He was given intensive Mapharside treatment which was discontinued because of a raised temperature on the fourth day, by which time he had received 780 mgm. On the fifth day he was drowsy. The drowsiness continued until he was unconscious. On the sixth day convulsions started and continued for three days. On the tenth day the convulsions became less but his condition deteriorated and he died.

At autopsy he was found to have active meningo-vascular syphilis and widespread acute cerebral petechial hæmorrhages, predominantly in the white matter.

The illustration (Fig. 111) shows the hæmorrhages in the internal capsules, infero-lateral to the lentiform nuclei and in the parietal and temporal white matter. *Microscopically* they are of ring type (Figs. 112 and 113), and are thought to be due to allergic sensitivity of the capillary endothelium to organic arsenicals (Russell, 1937).

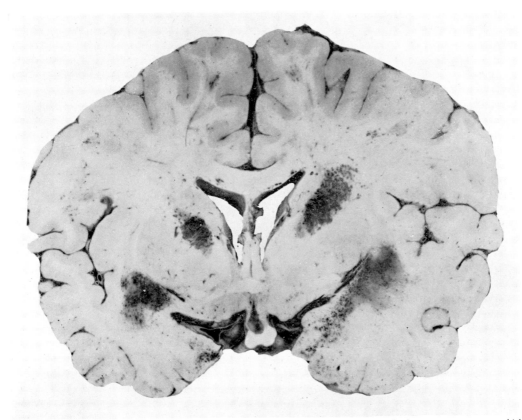

FIG. 111. *Coronal section of brain from a case of acute hæmorrhagic encephalitis (arsenical)* showing numerous petechial
hæmorrhages chiefly in the white matter.

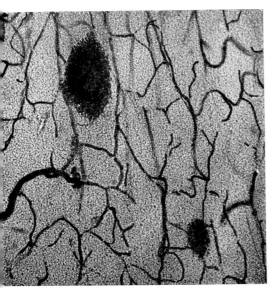

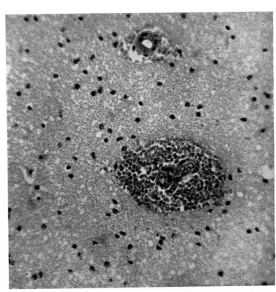

FIG. 112. *Vascular pattern in the cerebral white matter in arsenical encephalopathy,* showing hæmorrhages, often of ring or ball type, around the capillaries.
Pickworth preparation × 70.

FIG. 113. *Cerebral white matter from a case of arsenical encephalopathy,* showing the perivascular hæmorrhage and the hyaline degeneration or necrosis of the vessel walls.
Hæmalum and Eosin × 250.

CARBON MONOXIDE POISONING

Carbon monoxide produces its effects by anoxæmia. It changes the hæmoglobin of the red blood corpuscles into carboxyhæmoglobin, which is a stable substance and will not give up its oxygen for tissue metabolism.

For some, as yet uncertain, reason it usually exerts its main effects upon the globus pallidus, producing bilateral infarction in the antero-medial portion of the nucleus. This region is supplied only by branches of the anterior choroidal artery (a long slender artery). In a case dying shortly after exposure, the characteristic lesions in the globus pallidus are hardly visible to the naked eye (Fig. 114), but they should be clearly apparent in the brain of a person dying four or five days after exposure. Sometimes the cerebral white matter is severely affected (Figs. 115 and 118).

Fig. 118 illustrates the changes found in the brain of a patient in whom carbon monoxide poisoning was followed by severe amentia, associated with extensive damage to the cerebral white matter.

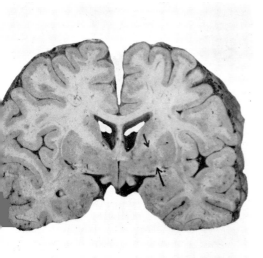

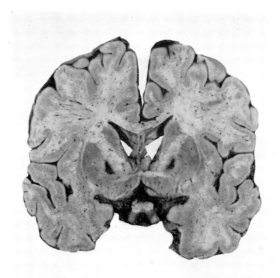

114. *Coronal section of brain from a man who gassed himself* *and a half days before death.* There was bilateral early *ening* of the globus pallidus (arrows). This is not easy to *macroscopically*, and consists chiefly of a loss of clear margin to the nucleus.

FIG. 115. *Coronal section of brain from a man who gassed himself twice* : once, three years before death (note bilateral cystic infarcts in antero-medial globus pallidus) ; and, again, two days before death (note the numerous petechial hæmorrhages in the white matter).

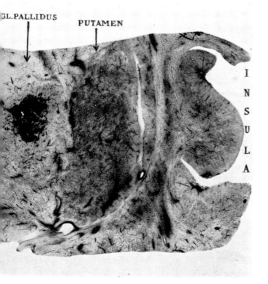

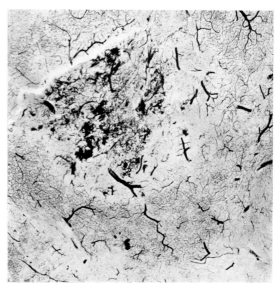

116. *Thick coronal section of the vascular lesion in a case of* *nt carbon monoxide poisoning*, showing the localization of the lesion to the upper medial portion of the anterior globus pallidus.

Pickworth preparation $\times$ 2.

FIG. 117. *Thick coronal section of basal ganglia from a case of recent carbon monoxide poisoning.* Note the focus in the globus pallidus showing intense vascular disturbance—dilatation of vessels, many perivascular (diapedetic) hæmorrhages. The parenchyma in the focus is necrotic.
Pickworth preparation $\times$ 7.

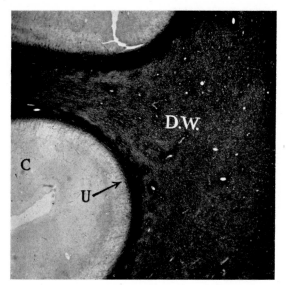

Fig. 118. *Cortex (C) and underlying white matter from a case of old carbon monoxide poisoning*, showing the extensive partial demyelination of the deep white matter (*D.W.*), and the relative sparing of the subsulcine arcuate or " U " fibres (*U*).
Myelin sheath stain × 11.

NUCLEAR JAUNDICE (KERNICTERUS)

Nuclear jaundice is found in 30 - 50 per cent. of babies dying from erythroblastosis fœtalis, which is due to an antigen-antibody reaction occurring in the fœtus, between the red blood corpuscles of the fœtus (Rh positive due to inheritance from the father) and the anti-Rh agglutinins of the Rh negative mother (who has been sensitized by the fœtus) which diffuse back across the placenta in the later months of pregnancy.

The bilaterally symmetrical nuclear jaundice is most marked in the basal nuclei, especially in the subthalamic nucleus (corpus Luysii) (Fig. 119), where the nerve cells are found to be degenerate and stained yellow. Nuclear jaundice, of a lesser degree, is also seen in the hippocampus, lenticular nucleus (especially globus pallidus), the dorso-medial nucleus of the thalamus, dentate nucleus, inferior olive and vestibular nuclei.

Greenfield (unpublished) notes that nuclear jaundice is most marked in the nuclei which are either mature or in process of becoming mature at birth, and he suggests that " There is at least a strong probability that the pathogenesis of kernicterus will be explained along the lines of antigen-antibody reactions occurring in relation to nerve cells, especially to those which have recently matured."

It should be noted that nuclear jaundice does not occur in babies who show generalized jaundice from some other cause (*e.g.*, congenital atresia of the bile duct).

The nervous system is not discoloured in jaundiced adults because of the impermeability of the blood brain barrier to the circulating pigment.

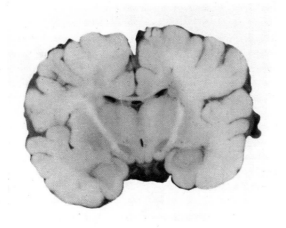

Specimen by courtesy of Dr Macgregor.

FIG. 119.   *Nuclear jaundice (kernicterus)* from a case of erythro-blastosis fœtalis. Note the yellowish colouration of the lentiform nucleus, thalamus, subthalamic body (corpus Luysii) (arrows), and cornu ammonis on each side.

HEPATO-LENTICULAR DEGENERATION
(WILSON'S DISEASE)

This is a condition in which there is an association of diffuse multilobular cirrhosis of the liver (Fig. 121) and bilateral degeneration of the lentiform nucleus, especially the putamen (Fig. 120). It is usually a familial condition, occurring in adolescence or early adult life and its pathogenesis is unknown.

Clinical Note.—A boy, the eldest of three children, with healthy parents and an uneventful family history, had jaundice and pale stools at the age of seven. Subsequently he had intermittent pyrexia, increasing difficulty in walking and developed tremor of his hands. When nine years and three months he was an obese, well-developed boy with bilateral gynæcomastia; the genitalia were normal for his age but pubic hair was present; he was unable to walk alone, and had marked tremor of the hands and legs. Wassermann's reaction of the blood was negative. His blood was Rhesus negative. He developed painful spasms in the arms, neck and legs, and these spasms became increasingly frequent. He lost the power of speech and died shortly afterwards.

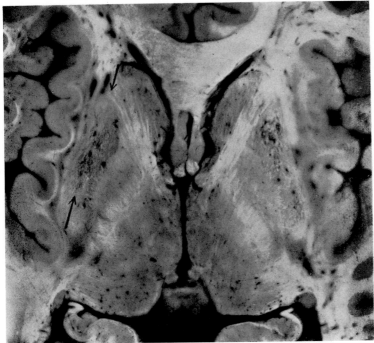

Specimen by courtesy of Dr Macgregor.

FIG. 120. *Horizontal section of brain in a case of hepato-lenticular degeneration*, showing the severe degeneration of each putamen (indicated on one side by arrows).

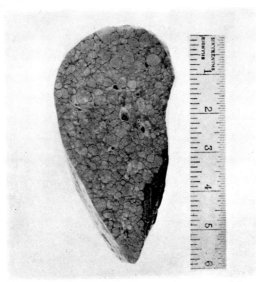

FIG. 121. *Parasagittal section of liver from a case of hepato-lenticular degeneration*, showing the diffuse nodular cirrhosis.

POLIOENCEPHALITIS HÆMORRHAGICA SUPERIOR
(WERNICKE'S ENCEPHALOPATHY)

The names given to this condition do not tell us its pathogenesis. The first indicates that it is a hæmorrhagic inflammation of the superior grey matter of the brain and the second only that it is a disease (*pathos*=suffering, disease) of the brain described by Wernicke.

In its acute form the condition displays itself to the naked eye as multiple small petechial hæmorrhages, invariably present in the corpora mamillaria (Figs. 122 and 123), commonly present in the grey matter bordering the 3rd ventricle and cerebral aqueduct and in the posterior corpora quadrigemina, less commonly present in the fornix, corpus striatum and cerebral cortex.

Microscopically the histological changes resemble the vascular reaction to some toxic substance, with vascular dilatation, stasis, and swelling of the endothelium of the capillaries (Figs. 124, 125 and 126).

Wernicke's encephalopathy is often associated with peripheral neuritis. Known to occur in alcoholics, it was shown by Campbell and Biggart (1939) to occur in other conditions, *e.g.*, gastric carcinoma, chronic dyspepsia, hyperemesis gravidarum. Wortis *et al.* (1942) showed that in such cases there was, in the blood, a raised fasting level of pyruvate (a step in the ladder of glucose metabolism which requires vitamin B1 for further metabolism). De Wardener and Lennox (1947), from observations on prisoners-of-war at Singapore, clinched the evidence that the condition was due to acute B1 (thiamine) deficiency. They found that, on a B1 deficient diet, the condition was usually precipitated by dysentery or diarrhœa, and was curable by thiamine injections. The earliest clinical features were those of anorexia, vomiting, nystagmus and emotional changes; only later came the classical semi-coma and the severe oculo-motor palsies.

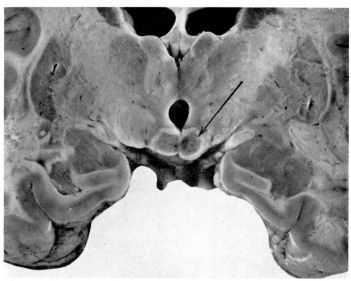

FIG. 122. *Coronal section of unfixed brain at the level of the corpora mamillaria, from a case of Wernicke's encephalopathy,* showing the petechial hæmorrhages in the corpora mamillaria (arrow).

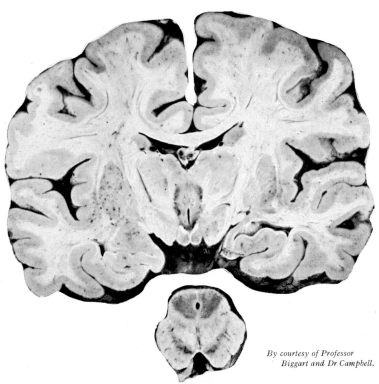

*By courtesy of Professor
Biggart and Dr Campbell.*

FIG. 123. *Coronal sections of cerebrum and midbrain, from a case of Wernicke's encephalopathy,* showing focal congestion and petechial hæmorrhages around the third ventricle, in the body of the fornix (just below the corpus callosum in the midline) and around the aqueduct extending into the inferior corpora quadrigemina (lower section).

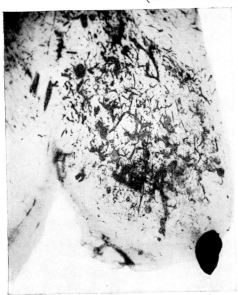

By courtesy of Professor Biggart and Dr Campbell.

FIG. 124. *Corpus mamillare from a case of Wernicke's encephalopathy*, showing the characteristic vascular disturbance—irregular dilatation of some vessels, partial occlusion of others, small petechial hæmorrhages. 250μ section. *Pickworth's benzidine stain* × 12.

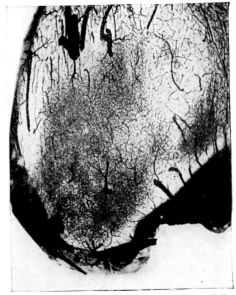

By courtesy of Professor Biggart and Dr Campbell.

FIG. 125. *Corpus mamillare from normal brain* showing passive congestion but no other lesion. 400μ section. For comparison with Fig. 124.

Pickworth preparation × 12.

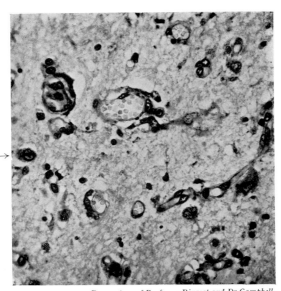

By courtesy of Professor Biggart and Dr Campbell.

FIG. 126. *Corpus mamillare from an acute case of Wernicke's encephalopathy*, showing vascular dilatation, endothelial hyperplasia and relative sparing of the nerve cells (arrow). *Nissl stain* × 300.

SUBACUTE COMBINED DEGENERATION OF THE CORD

This condition is usually associated with pernicious anæmia, but always with gastric achlorhydria. It is often accompanied by peripheral neuritis. The condition appears to be due to a nutritional deficiency.

Fig. 127 shows the typical foci of demyelination in the posterior and lateral white columns. The process is one of great swelling and degeneration of myelin sheaths and their contained axis cylinders. The disintegrated myelin is absorbed by phagocytes (Fig. 128), and carried away to the perivascular spaces, leaving large clear spaces (status spongiosus). For some unknown reason there is usually very little reparative gliosis (Fig. 129).

The degeneration in the posterior columns is the basis of the loss of touch, muscle, joint and vibration sense. The lateral column lesions, by interruption of the pyramidal tracts, give rise to extensor plantar responses. The loss of deep reflexes can be explained by the degeneration of either the peripheral nerves or the posterior column region, thus interrupting the afferent side of the reflex arc.

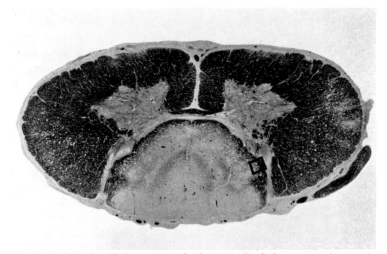

FIG. 127. *Cervical cord from a case of subacute combined degeneration*, showing the demyelination and " status spongiosus " in the posterior white columns and, to a lesser extent, in the lateral white columns. A region similar to that within the square appears in Fig. 128. *Weigert Pal* × 7.

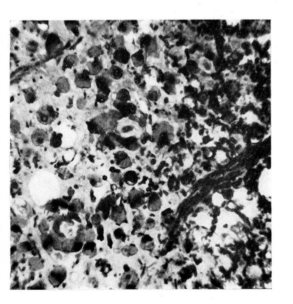

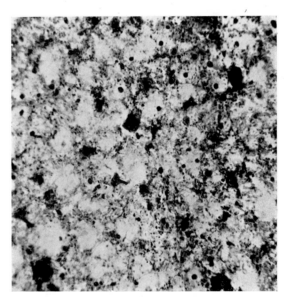

FIG. 128   FIG. 129

Fig. 128. *Posterior columns, from a region similar to that shown in the square in Fig. 127, from a case of subacute combined degeneration*, showing the vacuolation of the tissue (chiefly due to great swelling of the degenerating myelin sheaths) and the presence of fat (from broken down myelin) in phagocytes. Sometimes these compound granular cells can be seen within the ballooned out and degenerating myelin sheaths. This feature is not clearly seen here. *Myelin and Sharlach R. stain* × 200.

Fig. 129. *Transverse section of posterior white columns from a case of subacute combined degeneration*, stained for astrocytic fibres. It shows the very poor astrocytic response. Compare Figs 87-89. *Anderson's Victoria blue* × 200.

SECTION VI
DEGENERATIONS

SENILE DEMENTIA AND ALZHEIMER'S DISEASE

These two progressive degenerative conditions of the brain are histologically indistinguishable. Alzheimer's disease is usually found in persons below the age of 60 years, and senile dementia in persons above 60 years. Because of the widespread nature of the degenerative process there are well-marked symptoms of mental deterioration.

The changes consist of :—

(1) Widespread degeneration of the neurofibrils in many cortical nerve cells, with the formation of Alzheimer's neurofibrillary tangles (Fig. 132). Many of the degenerate nerve cells disappear.

(2) The presence of argyrophile (silver-loving) plaques in the grey matter (Fig. 132). One view of this change is that it represents a degeneration in the colloid substance of the brain. At first microglia are seen around and in the plaques (Fig. 133). Later the plaques become surrounded by astrocytes (Fig. 134).

Such widespread degeneration of nerve cells and their cell processes in the white matter, leads to atrophy of the brain, so that the external surface shows gyral atrophy (Fig. 131) and on section there is compensatory ventricular enlargement.

SENILE DEMENTIA AND ALZHEIMER'S DISEASE

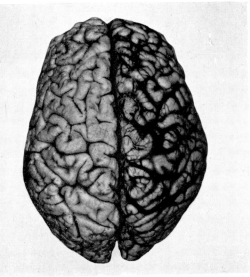

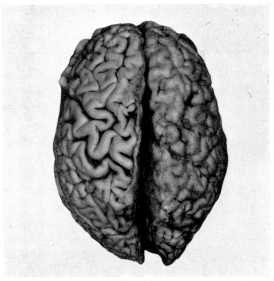

FIG. 130

FIG. 131

Fig. 130. *Normal cerebrum viewed from above, frontal poles at the top of the picture.* The arachnoid and cerebral vessels have been removed from the left hemisphere.

Fig. 131. *Cerebrum from a case of senile dementia viewed from above, frontal poles at the top of the picture.* The arachnoid and vessels have been removed from the left hemisphere. There is slight opacity of the leptomeninges due to slight fibrous tissue increase, usual in this condition. Note the marked widening of the sulci due to the cerebral atrophy.

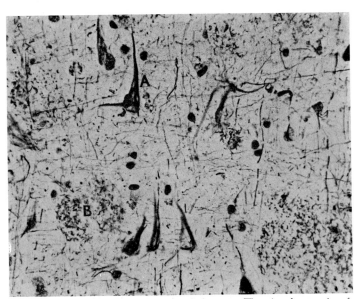

FIG. 132. *Cerebral cortex from a case of senile dementia.* There is a degeneration of the neurofibrils in many nerve cells with the formation of Alzheimer's neurofibrillary tangles (*A*). Compare Fig. 2. There are numerous argyrophile (silver-loving) plaques (*B*) between the nerve cells.
Von Braunmuhl's silver impregnation × 325.

93

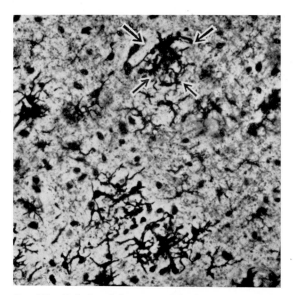

FIG. 133. *Early "senile" or argyrophile plaques, from an early case of senile dementia,* showing the numerous reactive microglia which appear to be attracted to the plaque. The arrows outline a plaque and its attendant microglia.
Silver impregnation for microglia × 150.

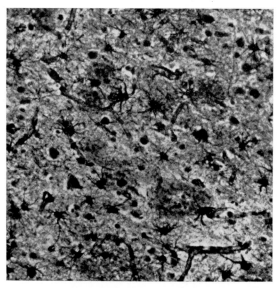

FIG. 134. *Cerebral cortex from a long-standing case of senile dementia,* showing the astrocytic reaction around the plaques.
Cajal's gold sublimate impregnation for astrocytes × 150.

95

PICK'S LOBAR ATROPHY

This progressive degenerative condition of the brain, with a predominantly lobar distribution, shows itself by bilateral atrophy of either the frontal or the temporal lobes (Fig. 136), and, less strikingly, on cut section, by an atrophy of the central white matter and often of the basal ganglia (Fig. 138). As a result of such widespread change there is marked mental deterioration.

Clinical Note (Fig. 136).—The patient was a man aged 66 years, with a ten years' history of loss of insight and disorientation. He could repeat only stereotyped phrases. His family had a history of arteriosclerosis and hypertension. He, however, did not show hypertension clinically nor was there evidence post-mortem.

Autopsy revealed marked atrophy of the anterior portions of both temporal lobes with fibrous thickening of the overlying pia-arachnoid. The atrophy affected the anterior portions of the superior, middle and inferior temporal gyri, the fusiform and hippocampal gyri. Frontal atrophy was present to a lesser degree. *Microscopically* the appearances were those of gradual neuronal atrophy, least marked in layer III, with replacement gliosis. There were no argyrophile plaques or neurofibrillary tangles and no evidence of vascular disease, thus excluding senile dementia and cerebral arteriosclerosis.

The condition should be distinguished microscopically :—

(1) From senile dementia and Alzheimer's disease by the focal lobar character of the atrophy.

(2) From atherosclerosis by the symmetrical character of the atrophy and by the absence of old cystic infarcts.

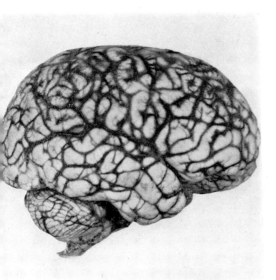

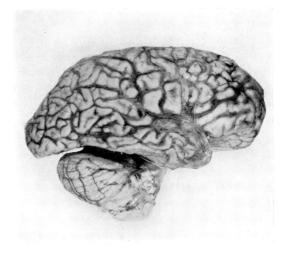

FIG. 136. *Lateral aspect of brain from a case of Pick's lobar atrophy*, showing the great atrophy of the temporal lobe. The left lobe was similarly affected.

FIG. 135. *Normal brain*—same scale as Fig. 136.

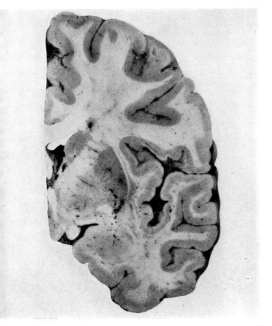

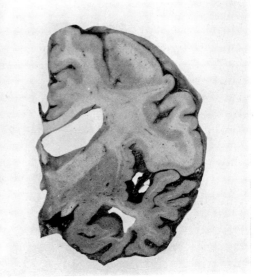

FIG. 138. *Coronal section of cerebral hemisphere at the level of the foramen of Monro, from a case of Pick's lobar atrophy*, showing the moderate generalized atrophy of the white matter and the marked focal atrophy of both white and grey matter of the temporal lobe. Note the compensatory internal hydrocephalus.

IG. 137. *Coronal section of normal cerebral hemisphere at the level of the foramen of Monro*—same scale as Fig. 138.

HUNTINGTON'S CHOREA

A diffuse degenerative process in the brain, with focal accentuation in the basal ganglia. The disease is hereditary and starts in adult life.

It consists of a diffuse neuronal atrophy in both cortex and basal ganglia, especially the caudate nucleus and the putamen (which are really one nucleus, being joined at their anterior ends and of similar cellular constitution). There are no specific microscopical changes, no senile plaques or neurofibrillary tangles. As a result of the neuronal atrophy, the brain shows widespread macroscopical atrophy of both cerebral white and grey matter (Figs. 140 and 142) with striking atrophy of the caudate and lentiform nuclei (Fig. 142). The clinical picture is thus a combination of extrapyramidal disturbance (chorea) due to the degeneration of the basal ganglia and of dementia due to the widespread cortical and white matter atrophy.

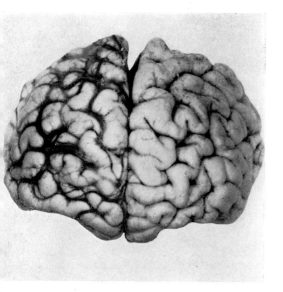

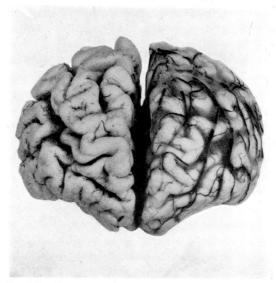

FIG. 139. *Normal frontal lobes.* On the right side of the picture the arachnoid and blood vessels have been removed from the cerebral hemisphere.

FIG. 140. *Frontal lobes from a case of Huntington's chorea.* On the left side of the picture the arachnoid and blood vessels have been removed from the cerebral hemisphere. Note the healthy leptomeninges and the deepening of the sulci due to the gross cerebral atrophy.

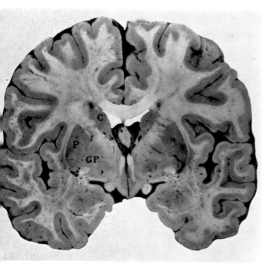

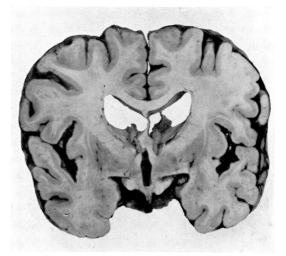

FIG. 141. *Coronal section of normal brain at the level of the fundibulum, on the same scale as Fig. 142.* Note the caudate nucleus (C), globus pallidus (GP), and the putamen (P).

FIG. 142. *Coronal section of brain, at the level of the infundibulum, from a case of Huntington's chorea,* showing the generalized cerebral atrophy, the marked atrophy of the caudate nucleus and, to a lesser extent, of the globus pallidus and putamen : and the resulting compensatory ventricular dilatation.

SYRINGOMYELIA

(Syrinx=a hollow pipe or tube, c.f., syringe)

Whilst a cavity in the cord can occur secondary to hæmorrhage or ischæmia, the type denoted by the term syringomyelia is one occurring characteristically, in either sex, at about the age of 20-30 years and manifesting itself clinically by dissociated anæsthesia, diminution or loss of deep reflexes and muscular atrophy with the frequent addition of spastic paraplegia and trophic disturbances.

The condition consists of a slowly progressive cavitation of the cord, usually starting in the cervical cord and spreading downwards. Sometimes the brainstem is involved (syringo-bulbia). The cavity varies in size and shape at various levels, and is rarely bilaterally symmetrical. It is bordered by astrocytic glial fibres and by a variable amount of collagen. Blood vessels, surrounded by astrocytic fibres, run across it. The central ependymal canal may or may not be involved, but the fibres of pain and temperature (and some of touch) are damaged as they cross in the anterior white commissure. The fibres of posture, vibratory sensation and touch, which run in the posterior white columns of the same side, escape (Fig. 143). This explains the ascending degeneration of the spinothalamic tracts and the dissociated sensory loss. Such a patient can burn himself painlessly with a cigarette : he can feel enough to hold it, but does not appreciate pain or temperature sensations.

The cavity in the cord enlarges and the surrounding cord substance degenerates. The crossed pyramidal tracts may be involved or the anterior horn cells may be damaged.

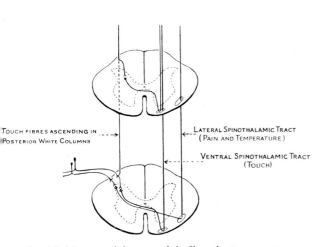

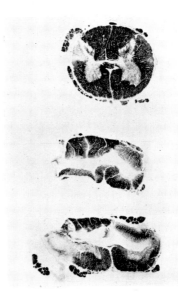

TOUCH FIBRES ASCENDING IN
POSTERIOR WHITE COLUMNS

LATERAL SPINOTHALAMIC TRACT
(PAIN AND TEMPERATURE)

VENTRAL SPINOTHALAMIC TRACT
(TOUCH)

FIG. 143. *Diagram of the course of the fibres of pain, temperature and touch in the spinal cord.* Note that touch has a double pathway, the more important of which is in the posterior columns, in common with that of vibration, joint and muscle sense. Thus a lesion in the region of the central canal (as in syringomyelia) will interrupt all the fibres of pain and temperature, but only a few of those of touch (dissociated anæsthesia).
(After Ranson).

FIG. 144. *Myelin preparations of the spinal cord in syringomyelia.* The upper section is from the lumbar cord, next the thoracic cord and the lowest section is from the cervical cord. Note the central cavitation increasing towards the cervical region. The secondary degeneration of the spinothalamic and spinocerebellar tracts is not well shown.
Weigert Pal stain.

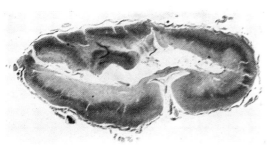

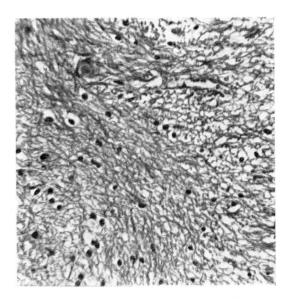

FIG. 145. *Cervical cord from a case of syringomyelia,* showing the marked central cavitation. On the upper wall (in the picture) of the cavity, to the left of centre, a more deeply stained astrocytic nodule projects into the lumen. This is not a common finding. Note that the cavity reaches the surface in the region of the left posterior horn. *Mallory's P.A.H.*

FIG. 146. *Higher power view of the mural nodule seen in Fig. 145,* showing the marked astrocytic overgrowth, with numerous glial fibres. The cavity is usually bordered by gliosis throughout, but in this case it was focally accentuated. This is not a common finding. *Mallory's P.A.H.* × 300.

FIG. 146

FRIEDREICH'S ATAXIA

This is a degeneration, most marked in the spinal cord, with a hereditary basis. Starting in childhood, the disease slowly progresses until it is fully developed.

The disease process is predominantly in the cord, which is atrophic in appearance and shows severe degeneration in the posterior and lateral white columns (Fig. 147), with marked reparative gliosis of a characteristic whorled pattern (Fig. 149). A minor degree of nerve cell degeneration may be present in the anterior and posterior grey columns. Russell (1946) has drawn attention to the subacute or chronic myocarditis which is often found at autopsy (Fig. 149).

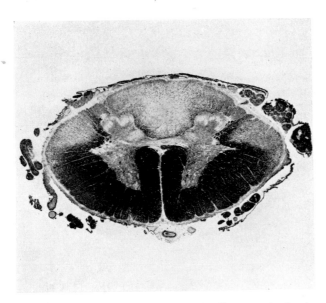

FIG. 147. *Thoracic cord from a case of Friedreich's ataxia,* showing the myelin loss from the posterior and lateral columns.
Weigert Pal stain × 8.

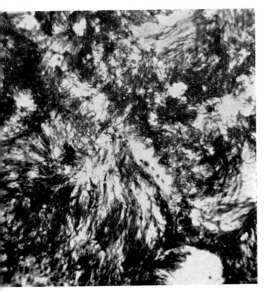

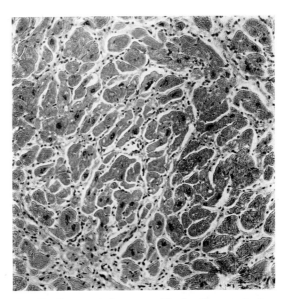

. 148. *Gliosis in the posterior columns, from a case of Fried-
h's ataxia,* showing the marked fibrous gliosis grouped in
rls or " tourbillons " in relation to the smaller blood vessels.
Anderson's Victoria blue × 200.

FIG. 149. *Heart muscle, from a case of Friedreich's ataxia,* showing
many large muscle fibres with large bizarre nuclei and cytoplasmic
vacuolation ; small atrophied fibres ; and slight interstitial
fibrosis and lymphocytic infiltration. *Hæmalum and Eosin* × 100.

MOTOR NEURONE DISEASE

Amyotrophic lateral sclerosis is a disease in which degeneration occurs in both the upper and lower motor neurones, namely, cortical neurones of the " pyramidal system," the motor nuclei of cranial nerves in the brain stem, the cells of the anterior horns of the spinal cord and the fibres which run peripherally from all these cells.

Progressive muscular atrophy is characterized by degeneration of the lower motor neurones. The cells and their processes which are affected are those in the anterior horns of the spinal cord and in the motor nuclei of the cranial nerves in the brainstem.

AMYOTROPHIC LATERAL SCLEROSIS

This degeneration, coming on in adult life and not hereditary, affects principally both the lower and upper motor neurones. The extent and level to which each is involved vary from case to case. In the spinal cord there is extensive degeneration of the anterior horn cells (Fig. 152) and of the pyramidal tracts ; but it is not a purely pyramidal tract degeneration, for, as Fig. 150 shows, there is extensive degeneration in most of the fibre tracts of the anterior and lateral white columns, though in many cases the spino-cerebellar tracts are spared. In well-marked cases the myelin picture in the spinal cord may be a " reversed tabes dorsalis " picture, the dark posterior columns standing out distinctly against the pale background of the rest of the cord.

In the brainstem the nuclei of the twelfth and eleventh cranial nerves, the nucleus ambiguus and the nucleus of the seventh cranial nerve often degenerate bilaterally, sometimes the motor nucleus of the fifth cranial nerve and the nuclei of the motor ocular nerves (third, fourth and sixth). In the cortex there may be degeneration of nerve cells in the motor cortex on the anterior lip of the central sulcus and in the precentral cortex.

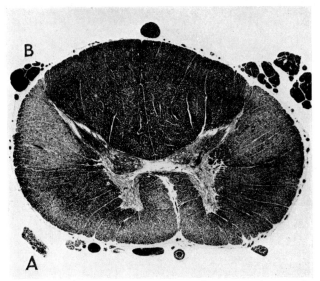

FIG. 150.   *Thoracic cord, myelin preparation, from a case of amyotrophic lateral sclerosis,* showing the widespread involvement of the anterior and lateral white columns (including the crossed pyramidal tracts) and the atrophy of the anterior grey columns.   As a result of the loss of anterior horn cells there is degeneration of the anterior spinal nerve root (*A*) which is seen to be paler than the healthy posterior nerve root (*B*).
Weigert Pal stain × 10.

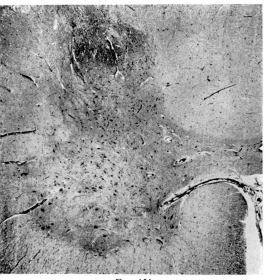

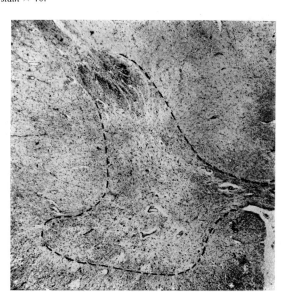

FIG. 151   FIG. 152

ig. 151.   *Normal lower cervical cord for comparison with Fig. 151.*   The anterior horn is in the lower part of the picture, the ventromedian ulcus on the right side of the picture.   Note the numerous anterior horn cells.   *Thionin stain* × 20.

ig. 152.   *Lower cervical cord from a case of amyotrophic lateral sclerosis,* showing the dotted outline of the anterior (lower) and posterior rey horns.   Note the loss of nerve cells from the atrophied anterior horn, and the increased number of small nuclei due to gliosis.   (Part f this prominence compared with Fig. 151 is artefact, due to the greater staining affinity of the nuclei in this section.)   *Thionin stain* × 20.

MOTOR NEURONE DISEASE
PROGRESSIVE MUSCULAR ATROPHY
(INFANTILE)

Generalized wasting and loss of tone in the voluntary muscles of infants, when not due to general diseases, such as rickets, may be due either to motor neurone disease (neuropathy) or to myopathy. In a **neuropathy,** degeneration occurs in the cells of the anterior horns of the spinal cord (sometimes of the lower cranial motor nuclei) and in the motor nerves which issue from them, with secondary degeneration of voluntary muscles. In a **myopathy** the degeneration is confined to the muscles. Confusion has arisen from the names given to the clinical manifestations, in infants, of these two different pathological conditions. Possibly Oppenheim (1900) may have included, under the name amyotonia congenita, cases both of the neuropathy previously described by Werdnig (1891) and Hoffmann (1893) and cases of the type of congenital myopathy later described by Batten (1903).

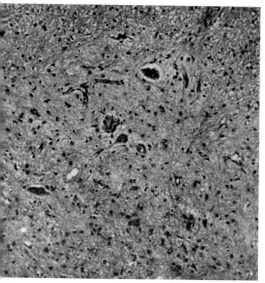

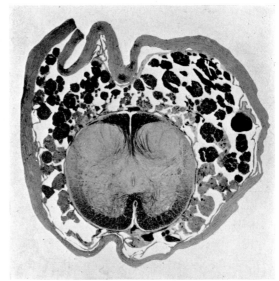

By courtesy of Drs Macleod and Macdonald.

Fig. 153

By courtesy of Drs Macleod and Macdonald.

Fig. 154

Fig. 153. *Anterior horn cells from the spinal cord of a case of Werdnig-Hoffmann's disease*, showing a reduction in the number of motor nerve cells and a compensatory astrocytic gliosis. Many of the remaining nerve cells are degenerating, one near the centre of the picture shows neuronophagia by microglia. *Mallory's P.A.H.* × 100.

Fig. 154. *Cauda equina from a case of Werdnig-Hoffmann's disease*, showing degeneration of the anterior nerve roots. These lie in the lower part of the picture. *Weigert Pal stain for myelin (stained black)* × 10.

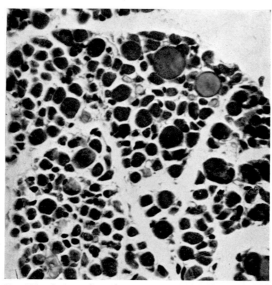

Fig. 155. *Intercostal muscle in transverse section, from a case of Werdnig-Hoffmann's disease*, showing degenerative changes in the muscle fibres similar to those following partial denervation. Some of the muscle fibres are of normal calibre, but many of them are abnormally slender with subsarcolemmal nuclear increase. A few fibres are swollen. *Hæmalum and Eosin* × 500.

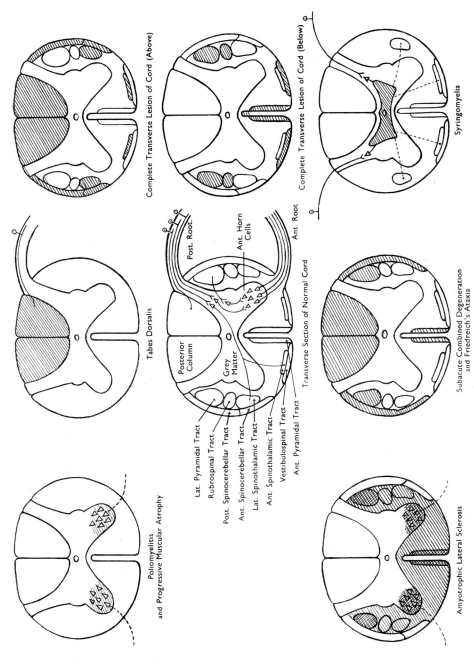

Complete Transverse Lesion of Cord (Above)

Complete Transverse Lesion of Cord (Below)

Syringomyelia

Tabes Dorsalis

Post. Root.

Ant. Horn Cells

Ant. Root

Posterior Column

Grey Matter

Transverse Section of Normal Cord

Subacute Combined Degeneration and Friedreich's Ataxia

Lat. Pyramidal Tract
Rubrospinal Tract
Post. Spinocerebellar Tract
Ant. Spinocerebellar Tract
Lat. Spinothalamic Tract
Ant. Spinothalamic Tract
Vestibulospinal Tract
Ant. Pyramidal Tract

Poliomyelitis and Progressive Muscular Atrophy

Amyotrophic Lateral Sclerosis

Fig. 156.   The shaded areas represent the affected regions in some of the commoner disease processes in the spinal cord.   The broken lines indicate interrupted nerve or fibre pathways above and below the lesions.

Note.—In Friedreich's ataxia the anterior pyramidal tracts are seldom involved : in subacute combined degeneration they are often involved.

SECTION VII

MECHANICAL TRAUMA

INTRODUCTION

The nervous system may be damaged either centrally or peripherally by mechanical trauma. The trauma may be direct : or may be indirect, mediated through the pressure of œdema or hæmorrhage around or into the nervous tissues.

EXTRADURAL INTRACRANIAL HÆMORRHAGE

Clinical Note (Figs. 157 and 158).—The patient was a boy, aged 15 years. He fell from a height on to a concrete floor and on admission was drowsy but conscious. The next day he became stuporose. His pulse rate began to fall. The right pupil became larger than the left and the plantar reflexes were extensor. Early next day he became comatose. Blood was not present in the cerebro-spinal fluid removed by lumbar puncture. That evening his temperature rose to 105° F. ; his pulse became very rapid and he died.

At autopsy there was a fracture of the skull and a tear of the right middle meningeal artery, with extradural hæmorrhage.

Figs. 157 and 158 show the brain and dura. On the surface of the dura is a large extradural clot in the temporo-parietal region—middle meningeal hæmorrhage. The brain is flattened below the hæmorrhage. In the brain-stem a small discrete hæmorrhage, 1 cm. in diameter, is seen in the superior part, on the right side of the midline. This is secondary to the acute rise of supratentorial pressure on the side of the extradural hæmorrhage (*see also* Fig. 197).

ACUTE SUBDURAL HÆMATOMA

This condition, which is not illustrated, must however be mentioned, because of its relative frequency in cases of head injuries in adults. The blood of the hæmatoma comes from torn surface vessels. Herniation of the hippocampal gyrus through the incisura tentorii, due to increased supratentorial intracranial pressure, is a common accompaniment of both acute subdural and extradural hæmorrhage. Patients with such conditions, unless treated, die within twenty-four hours to three days.

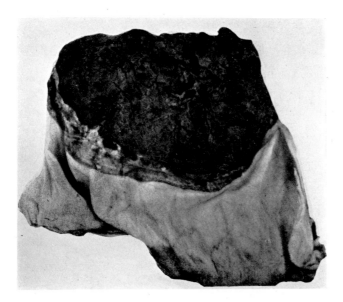

FIG. 157. *Outer surface of dura mater*, showing a large extradural hæmorrhage from torn middle meningeal vessels.

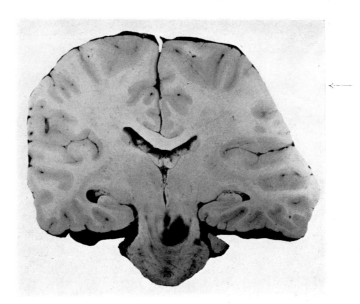

FIG. 158. *Coronal section of brain at the level of the substantia nigra in a case of extradural hæmorrhage*, showing (arrow) the flattening of the brain surface as a result of the hæmorrhage (Fig. 157). This case also shows a secondary brainstem hæmorrhage (often associated with a sudden unilateral rise of supratentorial pressure).

CHRONIC SUBDURAL HÆMATOMA

This condition may arise after severe, trifling or even forgotten trauma, and is thought to be due to rupture of a cerebral vein as it passes from the brain to the superior sagittal venous sinus (Fig. 159). Blood, with a variable amount of cerebro-spinal fluid, passes into the subdural space. A clot forms and adheres to the dura mater but not to the arachnoid membrane. The clot becomes organized, firstly on its outer or dural surface, then on its inner surface (Fig. 160). The more central part of the hæmorrhagic mass breaks down, producing a fluid of high osmotic pressure, which then attracts more fluid into its disintegrating substance, probably from the local blood vessels : thus the " tumour " increases in size. The condition may resolve or, by intermittent rupture of the thin-walled blood channels (Fig. 161) and further hæmorrhages, increase in severity. Amelioration of the patient's condition occurs in the interval between the hæmorrhages.

Since the process is usually slow, there may or may not be signs of increased intracranial pressure, but there will often be alteration of personality and headache. This possible combination of headache, raised intracranial pressure and alteration of personality may give rise to an erroneous diagnosis of frontal lobe tumour. Important points in differential diagnosis are said to be : (1) the profound lassitude ; (2) characteristic periods of remission of symptoms, in subdural hæmatoma.

Microscopically (Fig. 161) such a lesion shows the outer neo-membrane (the one close to the dura) to consist of a layer of moderately cellular fibrous tissue in which lie many thin-walled blood-containing channels. Amongst the fibrous tissue are many hæmosiderin-containing phagocytes (evidence of old hæmorrhage). Sometimes recent hæmorrhage can be seen to have occurred from one of the blood channels into the main body of the hæmatoma.

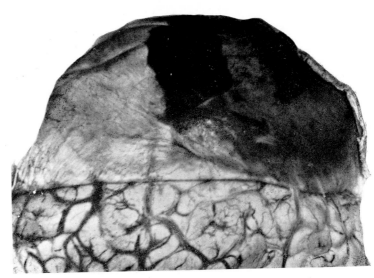

Venous lacuna.   Sup: long: sinus.   Diploic veins.

Direction of blow

To scalp.

DURA   DURA

CLOT

Sub·dural space.

BRAIN

Subarachnoid space.

Falx   Pia Mater

Cerebral vein.

By courtesy of Mr Rowbotham.

FIG. 159. *Chronic subdural hæmatoma.* Diagram showing the cerebral cortical veins running into the superior sagittal venous sinus. On the right one of these veins has been torn in its short extra-arachnoid course and a subdural hæmatoma has occurred.

FIG. 160. *Chronic subdural hæmatoma.* Male patient aged 54, no history of trauma, headache for two and a half months. Autopsy revealed bilateral fronto-parietal hæmatomata. In the specimen the dura has been elevated. On the right side the convex surface of the inner neo-membrane is seen ; centrally the hæmatoma has been cut across obliquely to show the massive clot ; on the left the hæmatoma has been scraped off the dura.

FIG. 161. *Subdural hæmatoma, three weeks after fracture of skull.* Section of the very vascular membrane which is growing from the dura (top of picture) down into the hæmatoma. Further hæmorrhage can easily occur from the large thin-walled blood channels.
Hæmalum and Eosin × 130.

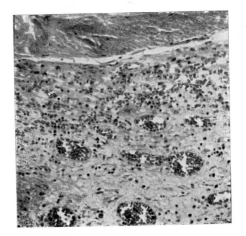

CEREBRAL TRAUMA

Injury to the head may be associated with injury to the brain in the form of (1) surface contusions and lacerations ; (2) injury to the deep structures.

Surface contusions and lacerations are found at autopsy to be most frequent in the supra-orbital frontal regions and around the temporal poles, regions where the brain lies upon dura covering bone with the most irregular surface. Contusions and lacerations are often more marked on the aspect of the brain which is remote from the site of impact of the blow (*contre-coup*) and less marked immediately below the site of impact of the blow (*coup*).

Many theories have been advanced to explain the mechanism of cerebral injury, but no single theory accounts for all the manifestations. Molecular disturbance of the nerve cells, and damage to blood vessels and nervous parenchyma produced by changes in velocity of the skull and its contents, are probably the most important effects of a severe cerebral injury. The main points arising from the observations of various writers are summarized below.

A. There are two components of a blunt head injury (Cairns, 1946) :—
  (1) The local injury beneath the site of the blow.
  (2) Distortions in parts of the brain remote from the blow, which depend on sudden changes of velocity of the head. Such changes of velocity may be rotational or linear in direction.

In (1) the scalp may be torn, the skull bends and may break, fragments may penetrate the brain. The brain may be bruised as well as torn.

In (2) when the head is made to rotate suddenly by a blow from a moving object or against a stationary object, the brain, not being rigidly attached to the skull, does not move simultaneously with it. The brain, being a highly incompressible substance in an enclosed space, makes the only kind of movement possible, namely a swirling movement (which may be of some magnitude and varies at different levels in the brain according to the blow and the way in which the brain is gripped or influenced by bony irregularities). The surface of the brain slides along inside the cranial cavity. Where the sliding movement occurs over rough surfaces the cortex will be more easily lacerated.

B. Holbourn (1943) has pointed out that :
(1) The rigidity of the skull is very great.
(2) Brain tissue is extremely incompressible.
(3) Brain has a very small modulus of rigidity, *i.e.*, it offers very little resistance to changes in shape compared to changes in size.

It is thus very susceptible to shear strains (the type of strain which occurs when a pack of cards is deformed from a neat rectangular pile to an oblique angled pile). Thus, in a head injury, damage to the brain will be most easily inflicted by forces producing shear strains, and not by those tending to compress the brain or deform the skull. Fig. 163 shows the variations in intensity of the shear strains, as estimated by Holbourn, in gelatin models subjected to rotation. The changes shown in these diagrams correspond in many ways to the distribution and intensity of brain damage found at autopsy in human cases of head injury. Note the tendency for the shear strains to be maximal at the site of a blow and directly opposite (Fig. 163 B), closely similar to the *coup* and *contre-coup* lesions in the human.

C. If the change in velocity of the head is in a linear direction, then the brain, having a greater mass than the skull, will accelerate or decelerate more slowly than the skull. On the side nearest the impinging force the brain will move closer to the skull : on the side remote from the impinging force the brain will tend to move away from the skull and a zone of negative pressure or suction will be produced. Small local veins subjected to this negative pressure will rupture, giving rise to hæmorrhage (*contre-coup lesion*) (Dott, 1944).

THE MECHANISM OF CEREBRAL INJURY BY ROTATION

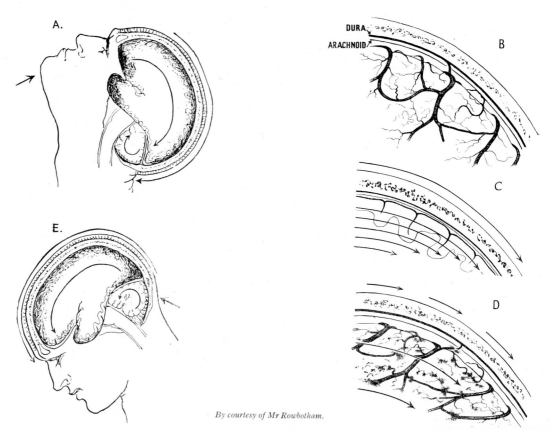

By courtesy of Mr Rowbotham.

FIG. 162. *Injury of the brain by rotation.* Whenever the head is struck by a force not directed along the line which passes through the centre of gravity of the head and the occipito-atlantoid joint (the fulcrum), it is caused to rotate. The skull necessarily takes the first impact of the blow and, since its mass is less than that of the brain, it accelerates faster than the brain. Then the brain is secondarily set into motion by the skull and particularly by projecting bony prominences and dural septa. The brain, having a greater mass than the skull, accelerates more slowly, at different rates at different depths, and shear strains are set up within the brain. The brain has a very low modulus of rigidity, *i.e.*, one portion of it will slide readily upon another. In closed injuries it is the shearing forces associated with deformity which cause the maximum damage to the cerebral tissues and tear the cerebral arteries and veins. (*A*) When a patient is struck on the chin the head is rotated backwards. (*B*), (*C*), (*D*) show the resulting deformity of the brain in relation to the vault of the skull. (*B*) shows the tissues at rest. One vein is shown running up into the dura (*e.g.*, to a venous sinus which is not shown). (*C*) The skull is now accelerating faster than the brain. The dura moves with the skull, the arachnoid with the brain. The brain is accelerating more slowly and at different rates at different depths (lengths of arrows indicate magnitude and direction of acceleration). The brain and pia-arachnoid are thus left behind relative to the skull and dura and shear strains are set up within the brain. (*D*) Towards the end of the rotation of the head. The skull is now decelerating and the results of the shear strains are to be seen in the numerous petechial hæmorrhages. The vein going to the dura has been torn in the sub-arachnoid space. (*E*) If a patient falls backwards and strikes his head on the ground, the head will be knocked forwards into an anterior rotation, the shearing strains in this case being in the opposite direction. Probably, in most accidents, the head is set into violent rotation about different axes at different phases of the infliction of the violence.

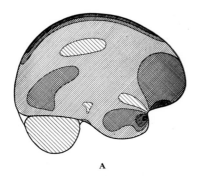

A

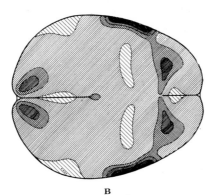

B

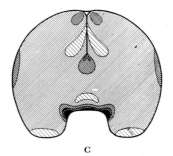

C

By courtesy of Dr Holbourn.

FIG. 163

Shear strains in gelatin models

A Intensity of the shear strains resulting from a forwards rotation caused by a blow on the occiput.

B Intensity of the shear strains due to a rotation in the horizontal plane caused by a blow near the upper jaw or temples.

C Intensity of the shear strains due to a rotation in the coronal plane caused by a blow above the ear.

Key.—Scale of maximum shear strain (=distortion) in arbitrary units of shear.   The units differ in the three diagrams.

CEREBRAL TRAUMA
Acute Lesions

The examples on the opposite page illustrate some of the early effects of cerebral trauma. Fig. 164 illustrates that, in head injuries, damage to the brain is more important than damage to the skull; furthermore, that unconsciousness and death may occur in the absence of gross cortical laceration. The mechanism of the injury to the brain has already been described. The hæmorrhage in the brainstem is obvious in Fig. 164. Fig. 166 illustrates the constant risk of massive intracerebral hæmorrhage which may, as here, be immediate, due to tearing of some large vein, or may suddenly develop some days after the accident, due to giving way of a vessel wall ("*Spät apoplexie*," Bollinger). Note how the hæmorrhage tracks in the line of the nerve fibre pathway, the natural line of cleavage.

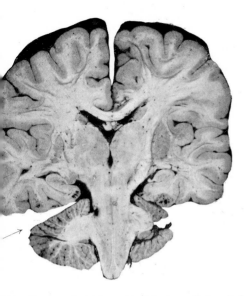

164. *Severe cerebral injury without fracture.* Patient died
e hours after receiving a severe blow on the jaw from the
ng ring of a 'bus wheel. Admitted unconscious with signs
ymptoms of brainstem injury. The brain is congested with
rous petechial hæmorrhages and contusions, especially in
the region of the incisura tentorii (arrow).

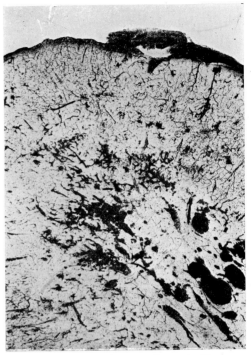

FIG. 165. *Severe cerebral injury.* Grey and white matter
from the hippocampus from the same case as Fig. 164,
showing dilated vessels and multiple capillary hæmorrhages.
Thick frozen section. Pickworth's benzidine method × 12.

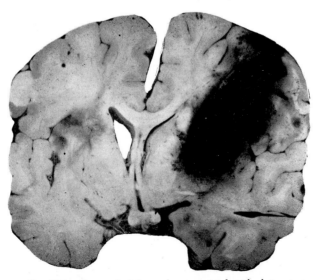

FIG. 166. *Intracerebral hæmorrhage associated with, but not
continuous with, compound fracture of orbit.* Massive venous
hæmorrhage which has tracked down from a subcortical vein
into the substance of the cerebral hemisphere. Death five days
after injury from secondary brainstem hæmorrhage due to
cerebral shift.

FOCAL EPILEPSY FOLLOWING TRAUMA

Following injury to brain tissue in which there is hæmorrhage and infarction (*e.g.*, traumatic laceration), the breakdown products are removed by histiocytes and repair is carried out by astrocytes and by connective tissue from blood vessels. The larger the region of necrotic cerebral tissue, the more connective tissue is found in the scar. When the damaged region is close to the pia or dura, the meninges take part in the process, and there result meningo-cerebral adhesions and a scar in which there is much connective tissue.

The secondary result is a slow contraction of the scar. This, in the appropriate region, may later give rise to focal epilepsy (Jacksonian). The exact cause of the epilepsy is not certain. It is probably due to vascular abnormality and variation at the edge of the scar. It has been shown at operation, under a local anæsthetic, that electrical stimulation applied to the region of such a scar results in an epileptiform seizure identical with that occurring spontaneously.

Figs. 167-169 show portions of the brain of a child who was knocked down by a lorry and sustained a compound fracture of the left frontal bone. This healed with adhesions between brain dura and skin. The infarcted cerebral tissue was absorbed (hence the cystic spaces in the frontal lobe) and a fibro-glial scar was produced. By contraction of this scar and by compensatory dilatation, the left lateral ventricle moved forwards and to the left (the so-called wandering ventricle). An adhesion had also developed between brain and dura in the left upper motor region.

Two and a half years after her accident she suddenly developed an epileptiform attack which passed into status epilepticus and she died.

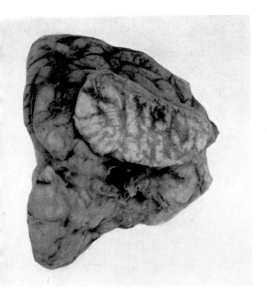

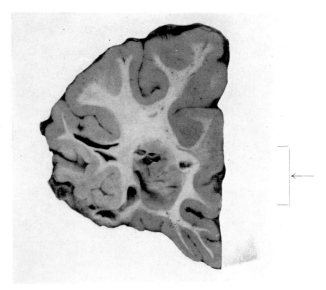

Fig. 167. *Anterior aspect of the left frontal lobe two and a half years after a compound fracture,* showing skin and subcutaneous tissues adherent, through an aperture in the skull (which has been removed) to scarred cerebral tissue. The skin is the raised mottled tissue in the central portion of the specimen. Below it lies the scarred cerebral tissue (around the black region).

Fig. 168. *Posterior aspect of frontal lobe shown in Fig.* 167. The cystic spaces represent the remains of the previously lacerated brain. Some of the cystic spaces communicate with the expanded tip of the anterior horn of the left lateral ventricle (lower right white matter : arrow).

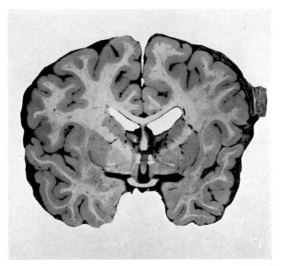

Fig. 169. *Coronal section of the same brain (as above) at the level of the optic chiasm, viewed from in front.* There is an adhesion between the dura and the brain in the left fronto-parietal region. Note the dilatation of the left lateral ventricle, secondary to the absorption of the damaged frontal tissue and the pull of the contracting frontal scar.

PYOGENIC INFECTION FOLLOWING CEREBRAL INJURY

In an open injury of the central nervous system there is always the risk of pyogenic infection. Organisms may be carried in by penetrating fragments or may grow down from the surface of the wound. Such a complication may occur shortly after the accident or may be delayed, often many years, as in this case (Fig. 170).

Clinical Note.—The patient was a man injured in the head by a shell splinter in 1916. He died in 1936. Two months before death he developed a large cerebral abscess, which was drained. His condition improved temporarily, but later he became drowsy and developed a left-sided hemiplegia.

At *autopsy* the dura was found adherent to the right temporal lobe. Pus was present in the basal cisterns.

Fig. 170 shows a small metallic fragment (arrow) surrounded by scar tissue which was continuous with the dura. Four abscesses of various ages are seen on the cut surface, three with fibrosed walls and one rupturing into the lateral ventricle. Pus was present in the ventricles.

Microscopically.—Abscesses of various ages were present—from an acute one which was really a spreading encephalitis to one which was enclosed by a thick layer of collagenous (fibrous) tissue surrounded by astrocytic gliosis and therefore of considerable duration.

Comment.—A small residual focus from the original wound had become active again or had been re-infected from the bloodstream. Spreading by retrograde venous thrombosis, daughter abscesses had formed. One had followed the unfortunate and common habit of abscesses and, enlarging chiefly in one direction, had ruptured into a ventricle.

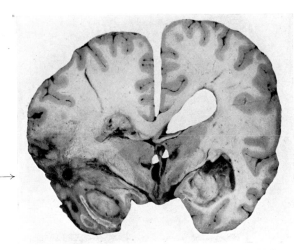

FIG. 170. *Coronal section of brain at the level of the infundibulum, showing the sequelæ of a penetrating wound of the brain.* The shell fragment (dark) is indicated by an arrow. Around it is old scar tissue. Below and medial are old surgically drained abscesses. Above and medial to it is a recent abscess which has ruptured into the ventricle. The right-sided ventricular dilatation is due to the obstructive communicating hydrocephalus caused by the space-occupying lesions in the left hemisphere.

SPINAL CORD INJURY

The bony and ligamentous tunnel, in which the spinal cord lies, is less rigid than the skull. In addition the cord has much less mass than the brain. Thus injuries of the spinal cord are unlikely to be due to movements within the substance of the cord, or between the cord and its surroundings, the result of relative differences in acceleration or deceleration. They are more likely to be due to nipping of the cord between displaced vertebræ, to stretching of the cord as a result of sudden flexion of the vertebral column, or to trauma to its blood vessels.

Œdema rather than hæmorrhage is the most prominent feature of cord injury. Hæmorrhage when it occurs is more common in the grey matter and is petechial rather than massive. In severe lesions the cord may be compressed or may be torn by forcible extension.

Fig. 172 illustrates the cord of a patient who fell twenty feet on to his shoulders. There was a forward dislocation of the fifth cervical vertebra upon the sixth cervical vertebra and the violent flexion of the spinal column meant that the cord was forcibly elongated (*cf.*, cord lies loosest in its canal in opisthotonos). This elongation tore many of the fibres in the cord, and there was hæmorrhage from the vessels. Secondary thrombosis added to the severity of the lesion.

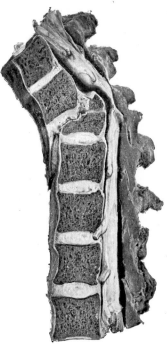

FIG. 171. *Injury to the spinal cord caused by a fracture of the lower thoracic spine. The spinal cord is both elongated and crushed. This is a more severe injury than that described in the text.*

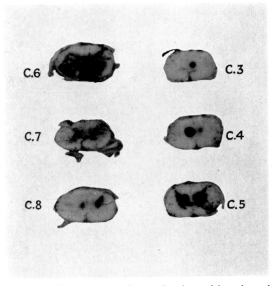

FIG. 172. *Severe injury to the spinal cord caused by a forward dislocation of C5 upon C6 vertebra (see text). Note the swelling of and hæmorrhage into the cord, more marked in the grey matter. The great linear extent of the lesion is due to the forcible elongation of the cord which accompanied the acute hyperflexion of the spine.*

PERIPHERAL NERVE INJURY

If a peripheral nerve is divided, the part below the lesion will degenerate, the cut end above the lesion will sprout new nerve fibres.

The degeneration below the lesion takes the form of disintegration of the axis cylinder and myelin sheath and removal of the products of degeneration by phagocytes. The space now left in the neurilemmal tubes becomes filled by proliferated Schwann cells, which sprout out of the ends of the severed tubes to form a " glioma " (Fig. 173).

The nerve above the lesion is still in continuity with its nerve cell, so that it lives and is able to regenerate. There is sufficient intraneural pressure in the axon so that axis cylinder substance begins to flow out slowly like a viscid fluid. At the same time there is an outgrowth of connective tissue and of Schwann cells to form a " neuroma " (Fig. 173). At first the outgrowths of axis cylinder substance are unmyelinated but in time they acquire a myelin sheath. If they can find their way into the distal stump they will grow down it (Figs. 175-177), and may eventually re-innervate the distal structures. If they do not find the distal stump they will interweave with each other and form a " neuroma " (Fig. 174). (*See also* Young, 1942).

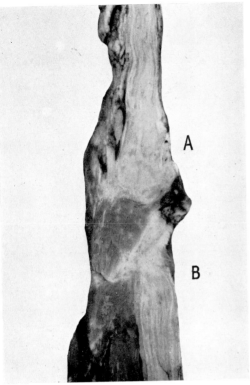

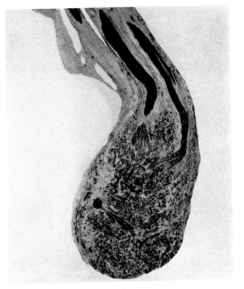

FIG. 174. *Longitudinal section of a digital nerve completely divided six months previously, removed because of pain on pressure (" trigger spot "), showing the " neuroma " composed of fine axis cylinders (now myelinated), of connective tissue and of Schwann cells.   Myelin stain × 10.*

FIG. 173. *Longitudinal section of sciatic nerve, completely divided by a shell splinter two months previously, showing the " neuroma " on the proximal stump (A) and the " glioma " of Schwann cells which has grown up from the distal stump (B). Muscle and scar tissue separate the stumps.*

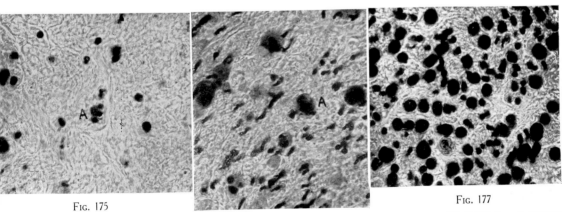

FIG. 175

FIG. 176

FIG. 177

By courtesy of The British Journal of Surgery.

FIGS. 175, 176 and 177. *The distal portions of interrupted regenerating nerves after varying periods of time.* At first the Schwann tubes contain only a little degenerate myelin (e.g. (A), Fig. 175). Then the axis cylinders grow down and become myelinated. At first these myelinated fibres are thin (Fig. 176) and unable to transmit nerve impulses properly. Myelin debris is still present ((A), Fig. 176). Later, with all myelin debris removed, both axis cylinders and myelin sheaths increase in calibre (Fig. 177) and become mature enough to function properly, provided that they have functioning end-organs.
    T. S. Myelin sheath stain × 280.

THE EFFECTS OF DENERVATION UPON MUSCLE

Figs. 178-181 illustrate the effects of denervation upon muscle.

Denervated muscle shows diminution in bulk, due in general to atrophy of the muscle fibres. Most of the fibres become more slender (Figs. 179 and 180) and eventually break up into short lengths or round up into spherical masses (Fig. 181). The subsarcolemmal nuclei appear to increase in number and may lie side by side in longitudinally orientated rows, or, in long denervated muscles, may be clumped together in groups ((A), Fig. 181). The sarcoplasm of denervated muscle retains its cross striation to a surprising extent. Connective tissue increase between the fibres does occur, but much of the increase may be more apparent than real, due to bunching together of pre-existent connective tissue.

Some muscle fibres break away from this process of gradual atrophy. They swell up and show vacuolar or granular degeneration of the cytoplasm (lowest fibre, Fig. 180) before they disappear.

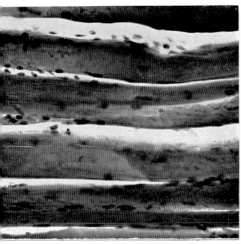

By courtesy of The Edinburgh Medical Journal.

FIG. 178. *Normal hypothenar muscle*, showing the fibre calibre, the cross striation and the nuclei. The nuclei, which appear to be within or very near the surface of the muscle fibres, are the nuclei of the sarcoplasm (subsarcolemmal nuclei, often, probably wrongly, called sarcolemmal nuclei). The nuclei between, or on the surface of, the muscle fibres are those of the capillaries and of the connective tissue of the fibrous endomysial sheaths of the individual muscle fibres. *This and the following three specimens were cut frozen at 18μ, stained Hæmalum and Eosin and are × 250.*

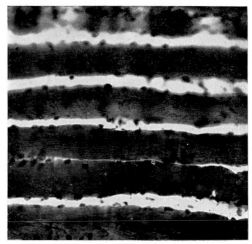

By courtesy of The Edinburgh Medical Journal.

FIG. 179. *Forearm muscle in longitudinal section, four months after complete denervation,* showing the diminution in calibre, partial loss of cross striation (the degree of this change is over-emphasized in the picture), and increase of subsarcolemmal nuclei. There is no fibrous tissue increase.

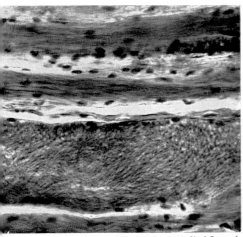

By courtesy of The Edinburgh Medical Journal.

FIG. 180. *Deltoid muscle two years after denervation.* Many of the denervated muscle fibres show a marked diminution in calibre with some loss of cross striation and an increased number of subsarcolemmal nuclei. One muscle fibre is swollen and is undergoing "granular degeneration" with disintegration of its fibrillar content. There is a slight increase of connective tissue between the muscle fibres.

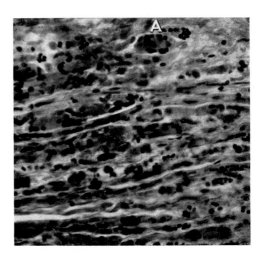

FIG. 181. *Leg muscle denervated twenty-one years,* showing the gross atrophy of the muscle fibres, some of which still retain cross striation. The fibres have become either shorter and slimmer or have rounded up into spherical masses (*A*). The subsarcolemmal nuclei are increased in number and give a very characteristic appearance to the spherical forms (*A*). Connective tissue is increased between the fibres.

REINNERVATION OF MUSCLE

The process of reinnervation of muscle depends greatly upon the length of time which has elapsed before the returning fibres reach the muscle. If the interval between denervation and reinnervation is short, the end result may be indistinguishable from normal. If the delay is long the axon will have difficulty in reaching the old end-plate. It will then leave its neurilemmal tube and wander about between the muscle fibres in an attempt to reform a physiological or anatomical contact with them (Figs. 182-185) (Gutmann and Young, 1944).

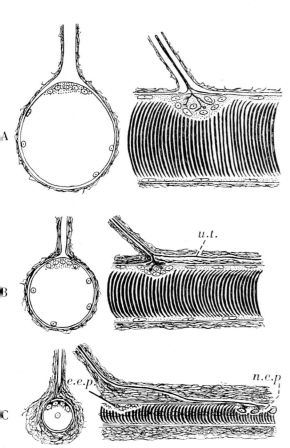

FIG. 182. *Diagram to show changes in relation of Schwann tube to muscle fibre as a result of progressive atrophy and fibrosis.* On the left the condition as seen in transverse section before innervation; on the right the result produced when the fibres return (seen in longitudinal section). *A.* Recent case. Very little atrophy, space above the end plate large, returning fibres able to branch in the old plate. *B.* Later case. Space restricted by fibrosis, part of the stream escapes to form an ultraterminal fibre (*u.t.*). *C.* Late case. End of tube closed by fibrosis and connection with old plate broken. Axoplasm wanders out to form a new end plate (*n.e.p.*).

Note. Schwann tube = neurilemmal sheath.

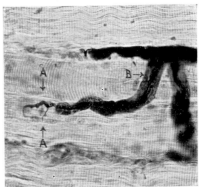

FIG. 183. *Normal motor ending (A) in muscle.* Note the myelin sheath (*B*) surrounding the axis cylinder as far as the end plate. *Axis cylinder stain* × 265.

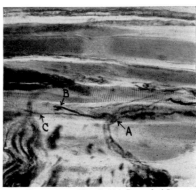

FIG. 184. *Regenerating nerve ending in muscle.* The axon has grown in from the right (*A*) and has formed a small end organ at (*B*). A portion of the axon has escaped from the neurilemma with the formation of an ultraterminal fibre (*C*). Compare Fig. 182 (*B*). × 265.

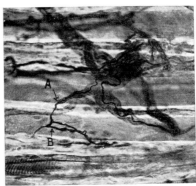

FIG. 185. *Regenerating nerve ending in muscle.* The regenerating axon has grown out from its old neurilemma (*A*) and formed a nerve network (*B*) between the muscle fibres. × 265.

SECTION VIII
HYDROCEPHALUS AND DISPLACEMENT
CEREBRO-SPINAL FLUID

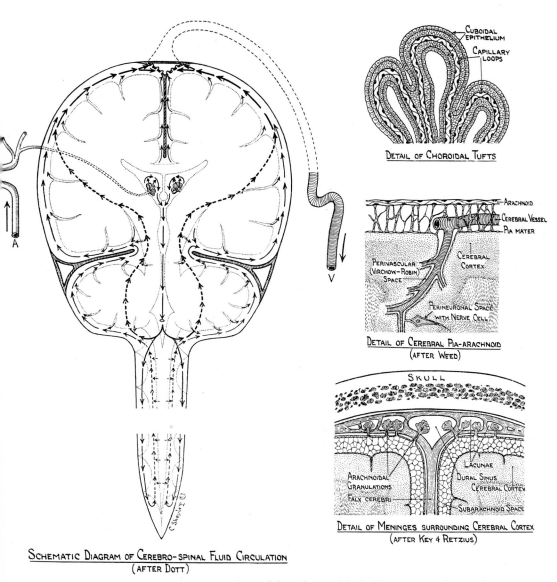

CUBOIDAL EPITHELIUM

CAPILLARY LOOPS

DETAIL OF CHOROIDAL TUFTS

ARACHNOID

CEREBRAL VESSEL

PIA MATER

PERIVASCULAR (VIRCHOW-ROBIN) SPACE

CEREBRAL CORTEX

PERINEURONAL SPACE WITH NERVE CELL

DETAIL OF CEREBRAL PIA-ARACHNOID
(AFTER WEED)

SKULL

ARACHNOIDAL GRANULATIONS

FALX CEREBRI

LACUNAE

DURAL SINUS

CEREBRAL CORTEX

SUBARACHNOID SPACE

DETAIL OF MENINGES SURROUNDING CEREBRAL CORTEX
(AFTER KEY & RETZIUS)

SCHEMATIC DIAGRAM OF CEREBRO-SPINAL FLUID CIRCULATION
(AFTER DOTT)

FIG. 186. *Diagrams to illustrate the normal circulation of the cerebro-spinal fluid.* (The perineuronal space, shown in the middle right-hand picture, is considered by most authorities to be an artefact.) The choroid plexuses in the 4th ventricle have been omitted, for the sake of clarity.

133

HYDROCEPHALUS

Hydrocephalus (an increased amount of cerebro-spinal fluid within the skull) may be :—

(1) **Compensatory.** — Secondary to gyral or cerebral atrophy, usually both internal and external.

(2) **Obstructive.**—Due to blockage of the cerebro-spinal fluid pathway between its point of origin from the choroid plexuses and its point of passage through the arachnoidal granulations into the venous sinuses. If the block is rostral to the apertures in the 4th ventricle it is called NON-COMMUNICATING. If the pathway of the cerebro-spinal fluid is not blocked until the fluid has passed out of the 4th ventricle to the outside of the brain, *e.g.*, obliteration of the basal cisterns at the midbrain level by organized meningococcal leptomeningitis, then it is called COMMUNICATING hydrocephalus.

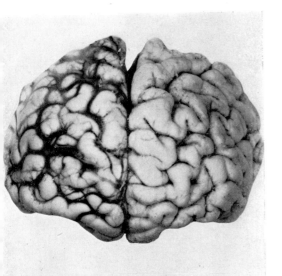

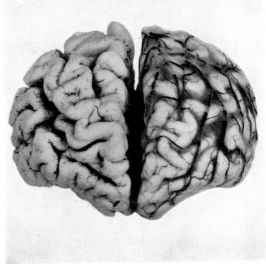

FIG. 187. *Normal frontal lobes.* The arachnoid and blood vessels are present on the left side of the picture ; they have been removed on the right side.

FIG. 188. *Frontal lobes, compensatory hydrocephalus* due to atrophy of the brain in Huntington's chorea. The arachnoid has been removed on the left side of the picture. Note the deepened sulci. (*See also* Figs. 138, 142.)

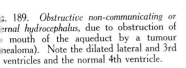

FIG. 189. *Obstructive non-communicating or internal hydrocephalus,* due to obstruction of the mouth of the aqueduct by a tumour (pinealoma). Note the dilated lateral and 3rd ventricles and the normal 4th ventricle.

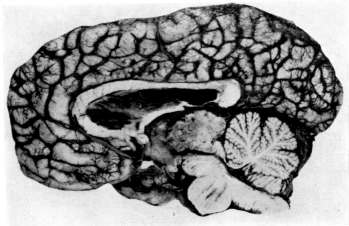

FIG. 190. *Obstructive communicating hydrocephalus,* due to blockage, by adhesions following meningococceal meningitis, of the cerebrospinal fluid pathway around the midbrain. Note that all the ventricles are dilated. (See also Figs. 194 and 197.)

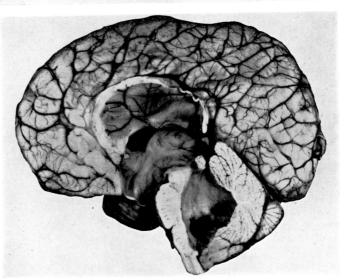

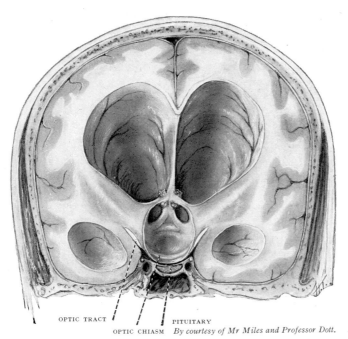

OPTIC TRACT   PITUITARY
OPTIC CHIASM   *By courtesy of Mr Miles and Professor Dott.*

FIG. 191. *The effects on the brain of chronic internal obstructive hydrocephalus.*
Note the thinning of the white matter, due to interference with its blood
supply (more vulnerable than that of the cortex) by the raised intracranial
pressure. The 3rd ventricle is distended, its floor ballooned out and thinned.
Hypothalmic nerve centres are damaged thereby and the optic chiasm is
stretched. The pituitary gland is directly compressed. The mechanism
of damage is again that of obstruction of the blood flow.

EFFECTS OF INTRACRANIAL SPACE-OCCUPYING LESIONS

Much of the clinical effect of intracranial space-occupying lesions is produced by (1) local destruction; (2) shift. Shift may be divided into lateral shift and downward shift (though the effect is usually due to a combination of the two).

LATERAL SHIFT

This leads to (1) distortion of the ventricular system, possibly with obstruction to the circulation of the cerebro-spinal fluid. (2) If anterior, there may be considerable distortion of, and interference with, the blood supply of the basal ganglia and hypothalamus (Fig. 193). (3) The cerebral peduncle on the side opposite to the space-occupying lesion may be pressed against the free edge of the tentorium cerebelli. If this displacement occurs quickly, the tentorium does not yield and the peduncle is damaged (Figs. 192 and 194). Clinical features resulting from damage to the peduncle may be misinterpreted, as being due to a space-occupying lesion on the side of the brain opposite to that in which the space-occupying lesion is really present.

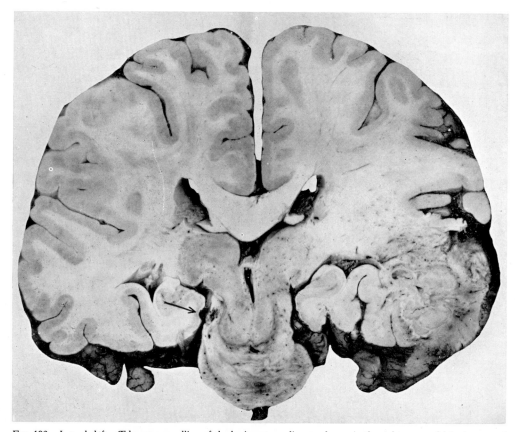

Fig. 192. *Lateral shift.* Œdematous swelling of the brain surrounding an abscess in the right temporal lobe has caused a rapid displacement of the basal part of the brain to the left. The arrow shows where the left cerebral peduncle has been damaged by pressure against the free edge of the dura of the tentorium cerebelli.

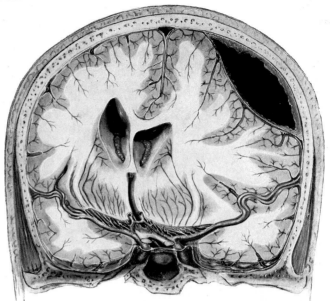

Fig. 193. *Lateral shift*. A space-occupying lesion (chronic subdural hæmatoma) is present on the right side of the picture. It has caused displacement of the brain to the opposite side. Note the displacement of part of the brain beneath the arch of the falx cerebri. Note the small perforating vessels which supply the basal nuclear region. They are relatively fixed to the base of the skull by the main arterial trunks. The shift of the brain puts tension on these vessels.

By courtesy of Mr Miles and Professor Dott.

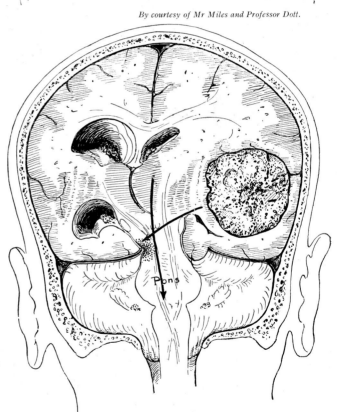

Fig. 194. *Combined lateral and downward shift (semi-diagrammatic)*. Coronal section of brain viewed from in front. A tumour is present in the left fore-brain compartment. The arrows indicate the direction of the resulting displacement. The whole brainstem is pushed downwards towards foramen magnum. The lateral and downward displacement forces the (true) right crus against the adjacent edge of the incisura tentorii. It also forces part of the left hippocampal gyrus down through the incisura and thus the whole brainstem is compressed at this level. The cerebro-spinal fluid pathway is blocked by this tentorial impaction so that there is distension of the lateral and 3rd ventricles. This distension is not uniform because of the left-sided tumour.

By courtesy of Mr Miles and Professor Dott.

DOWNWARD SHIFT

The contents of the supratentorial compartment will be displaced through the incisura tentorii with resulting **tentorial herniation** of the hippocampus (Figs. 195 and 196), and the hind brain will be pushed through the foramen magnum with resulting **foraminal impaction** (Fig. 198).

The impaction of the hippocampus in the incisura tentorii will cause obstruction to the flow of cerebro-spinal fluid past the midbrain with obstructive hydrocephalus. The herniated uncus will compress the 3rd cranial nerve against the anterior part of the free edge of the tentorium cerebelli, against the portion which is attached to the posterior clinoid process. This leads to PARALYSIS OF THE 3RD NERVE (Fig. 195). If rapid (and unilateral) the displacement may lead to such distortion of the arteries of the upper brainstem that BRAINSTEM HÆMORRHAGE occurs (Fig. 197). The downward shift of the brainstem causes 6TH NERVE PALSY (Fig. 195). The herniation of the cerebellar tonsils into the foramen magnum and the squeezing together of the contents of the posterior fossa at that level, leads to obstruction of the apertures of the 4th ventricle with OBSTRUCTIVE HYDROCEPHALUS (Fig. 198).

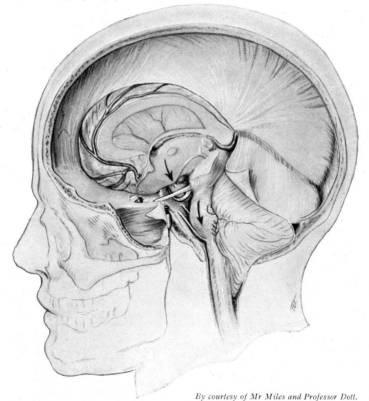

By courtesy of Mr Miles and Professor Dott.

FIG. 195. *Paresis of the 3rd and 6th cranial nerves by cerebral displacement.* A space-occupying lesion, not shown, is present in the right forebrain compartment. The hippocampal gyrus on the right side has been forced down through the incisura tentorii. The right 3rd nerve is pressed upon by this protrusion. The brainstem is dislocated downwards and the 6th nerve is subjected to angulation and to stretching.

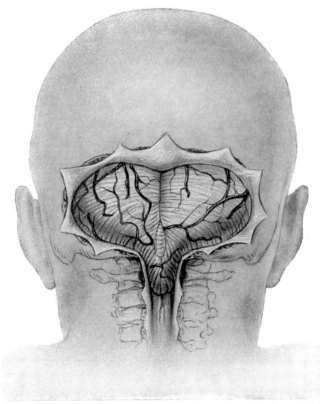

By courtesy of Mr Miles and Professor Dott.

FIG. 198. *Foraminal impaction or cerebellar coning.* The cerebellum and brainstem have shifted downwards and produced obstruction to the egress of cerebrospinal fluid from the 4th ventricle. This starts a vicious circle of obstructive hydrocephalus. By decompression alone the surgeon encourages the brainstem to rise and frees the exits from the 4th ventricle.

143

SECTION IX
TUMOURS

EFFECTS OF INTRACRANIAL TUMOURS

These may be local and/or general.

The **local symptoms** may be prominent due to tissue destruction (tumour of 8th nerve), or slight (diffuse astrocytoma which infiltrates but does not appreciably destroy). Local symptoms may be true (at the site of the tumour) or false (remote from the tumour). For example, a large tumour in the cerebral hemisphere pushes down the brainstem, the 6th nerve becomes stretched and bent acutely where it pierces the dura, its blood supply at this point is impaired and a false-localizing 6th nerve palsy develops.

The **general symptoms** are eventually common to nearly all cases, and are those of raised intracranial pressure, for intracranial tumours are growing within a bony container. As a rule the tumour also causes obstruction to the pathway of the cerebro-spinal fluid and the intracranial pressure rises. Clinically the classical result is (1) Papilloedema; (2) Vomiting; (3) Headache.

PAPILLŒDEMA results from obstruction to the venous return from the optic nerve region. The veins are obstructed as they leave the optic nerves and cross the subarachnoid space which ensheaths the optic nerves.

VOMITING is probably due to irritation of the medullary centres by interference with their blood supply.

HEADACHE is due either to stretching of the dura in the region of the venous sinuses, or to painful stimuli resulting from alterations in the calibre of blood vessels.

THE GLIOMATA

These are the commonest intracranial tumours. They are of many kinds, and the nomenclature is perhaps confusing. Bailey and Cushing (1926) classified them on an embryological basis, the tumour being called after the actual or hypothetical embryological cell which the tumour cell most closely resembled.

They may be considered as arising :—

(1) From " rests " or residues of undifferentiated cells left over from embryological development (*e.g.*, medulloblastoma).

(2) From neoplasia of adult cells already present (*e.g.*, astrocytoma).

(3) From neoplasia and dedifferentiation of adult cells (*e.g.*, glioblastoma multiforme).

Classes.	Relative Frequency.	Average duration of life after onset.	
Astrocytoma	37·0%	76 +	months
Glioblastoma multiforme	30·2%	12	,,
Medulloblastoma	12·6%	15	,,
Astroblastoma	5·1%	37 +	,,
Spongioblastoma polare	4·7%	46 +	,,
Oligodendroglioma	4·0%	66 +	,,
Ependymoma	3·7%	25 +	,,
Pinealoma	2·0%	18 +	,,
TOTAL	99·3%		

(After Cushing, 1932.)

Note that the astrocytoma is the most benign and the glioblastoma multiforme the most fatal.

Note also that the first three are the common ones, the others being much less frequent.

ASTROCYTOMA

A slow-growing, usually diffusely infiltrating, occasionally localized tumour occurring most commonly in the cerebral hemisphere in adults, in the cerebellum or pons in children. It frequently undergoes cystic degeneration. In adults it may, in some part, undergo malignant de-differentiation and become a glioblastoma multiforme.

Microscopically an astrocytoma shows the following characteristic features :—

(1) Uniform cell type and pattern, usually a meshwork of one kind of mature astrocyte (*e.g.*, protoplasmic, fibrillary or gemästete astrocyte).

(2) Very infrequent or no mitotic figures.

(3) No particular perivascular pattern.

(4) Cyst formation due to degeneration, but no large regions of necrosis.

(5) Fine thin-walled blood vessels, often probably those of the pre-existent normal nervous tissue.

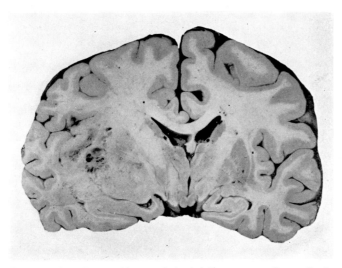

FIG. 199. *Coronal section of brain at the level of the corpora mamillaria.* On the left side of the picture there is a cystic astrocytoma in the basal ganglia. It is firm in consistence for it contains numerous glial fibrils. Note how ill-defined is the margin between brain and tumour. This is due to the infiltrating nature of the tumour. Note also the displacement of midline structures to the right.

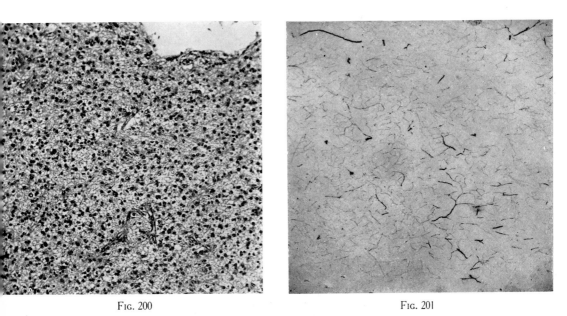

FIG. 200   FIG. 201

Fig. 200. *Portion of astrocytoma similar to that in Fig.* 199. The tumour is both cellular and vascular. It has a uniform cell pattern without perivascular arrangement. The cells resemble mature astrocytes. The blood vessels are small with thin healthy walls. At the top of the picture is one of the cystic cavities, surrounded by tumour cells, formed apparently by cytolysis of the astrocytes.
Mallory's P.A.H. × 100.

Fig. 201. *The vascular pattern of a typical astrocytoma,* showing its regularity. Compare with Fig. 204.
Thick frozen section. Pickworth benzidine preparation × 11.

GLIOBLASTOMA MULTIFORME

A common glioma in adults, usually occurring in the cerebral hemispheres. It is a rapidly growing destructive tumour; it does not infiltrate silently like an astrocytoma.

Fig. 203 shows the characteristic *microscopical picture* :—

(1) Cells of different shapes (pleomorphism) and different types ("multiforme"), *e.g.*, giant cells and primitive types of glial cells ("glioblast").

(2) Mitotic figures.

(3) Palisading around necrosis.

(4) Capillary endothelial hyperplasia. This is a non-specific reaction on the part of the endothelial cells of the capillaries and is associated with a slow blood circulation. It is found in other gliomata (*e.g.*, astroblastoma). The slow blood flow and the tendency to thrombosis explain the frequency of necrosis.

Figs. 203 and 204.

Fig. 203. *Glioblastoma multiforme (same magnification as Fig. 200)*, showing the characteristic variation in cell size and type, sometimes with multinucleated giant cells (top right corner); the palisading of cells around regions of necrosis ("wreath rosette," left side of picture); and the overgrowth of capillary endothelial cells (shown as a tangled mass of several vessels, bottom right corner). *Hæmalum and Eosin* × 100.

Fig. 204. *Glioblastoma multiforme, vascular pattern*, showing the large vascular spaces which are subject to thrombosis and hæmorrhage. There is a portion of "normal" cortex in the top right corner of the picture. Compare with Fig. 201. *Pickworth preparation* × 5.

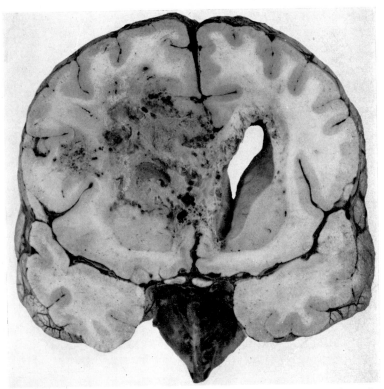

FIG. 202. *Coronal section of brain showing a glioblastoma multiforme.* It is a destructive tumour, with an ill-defined edge. It shows large blood vessels, yellow regions of necrosis and cystic spaces filled with thick greenish fluid as well as the, usually peripheral, reddish fleshy tumour.

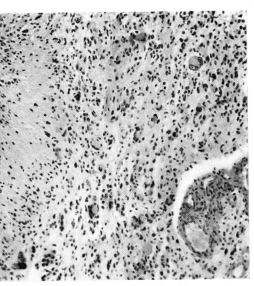

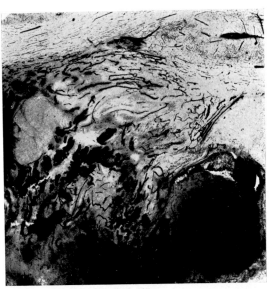

FIG. 203

FIG. 204

MEDULLOBLASTOMA

Next to the astrocytoma this is the commonest tumour of childhood. It almost invariably arises in the cerebellum, is very radiosensitive, but has the unfortunate habit of " seeding " readily in the subarachnoid space of the cord.

Fig. 205 shows such a tumour, arising in the superior vermis of the cerebellum, with obstruction of the cerebro-spinal fluid pathway. " Seeding " of a similar tumour in the spinal subarachnoid space is shown in Fig. 206.

Microscopically (Fig. 207) such a tumour shows the following features :—

(1) Very cellular.

(2) Cells closely packed, little cytoplasm, deeply staining nuclei, no perivascular pattern.

(3) Many mitoses.

(4) Fine blood vessels, no large regions of necroses.

The type cell is supposed to be akin to a hypothetical multipotential cell of the primitive neural tube—the medulloblast. This tumour is closely akin to the ependymoblastoma.

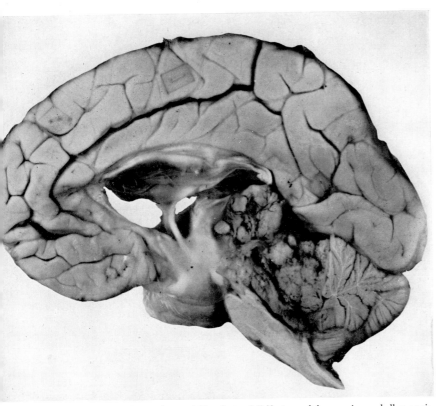

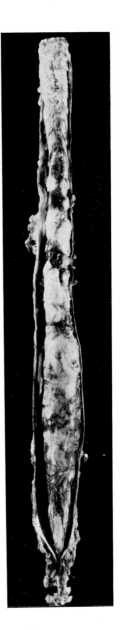

5. 205. *Median sagittal section of brain from a child with a medulloblastoma* of the superior cerebellar vermis, wing the tumour filling the 4th ventricle and causing obstructive internal hydrocephalus. It is soft, greyish and friable (for it contains no fibrillar material.)

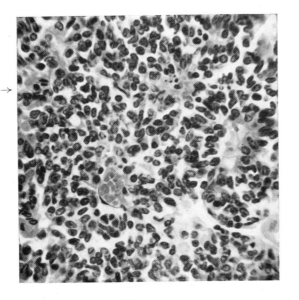

5. 207. *Medulloblastoma* show-
the highly cellular, vascular
nour. The cells are small,
ngated, with little cytoplasm
d hyperchromatic nuclei, often
mitosis (5 mm. in from edge of
ture at arrow), arranged in
d masses or in pseudo-rosettes.
ch a rosette, with its centre
ed with acidophile cell pro-
ses and debris, is seen at 1
lock from the centre of the
ture. Note the thin-walled
ssel at 7 o'clock from centre.
Hæmalum and Eosin × 350.

FIG. 206. *Spinal cord of
a child with a cerebellar
medulloblastoma,* showing
the numerous tumour seed-
lings which have floated
down in the cerebro-spinal
fluid, implanted them-
selves, especially in the
region of the cauda equina,
and grown into a massive
coating for the cord.

EPENDYMOMA AND CHOROIDAL PAPILLOMA

These two tumour types are closely related, for the choroidal plexuses are formed embryologically by an invagination, by vascular processes, of the ependymal roof of the brain. The ependymoma is the commonest tumour in the spinal cord. In the brain it is found close to or in the wall of a ventricle.

The diagnosis of an **ependymoma** depends greatly upon the pattern assumed by the tumour cells (Fig. 209), which may be either or both :—

(1) The formation of canals lined by cubical epithelium.

(2) The perivascular arrangement of spindle-shaped cells (ependymal spongioblasts).

The blood vessels are thin-walled and numerous.

On microscopical examination a **choroidal papilloma** is seen to have a papillary arrangement and to be formed of numerous fine thin-walled blood vessels covered by cubical or columnar epithelium. Choroidal papillomas have an unfortunate habit of " seeding " down the spinal subarachnoid space.

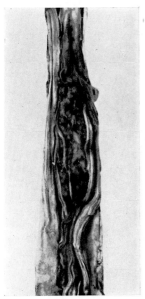

FIG. 208. *Lumbosacral cord and cauda equina, with a massive ependymoma,* growing slowly in the cauda equina.

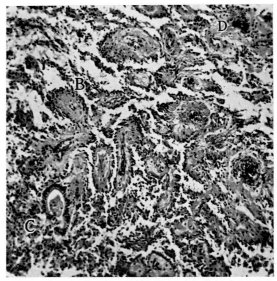

FIG. 209. *Ependymoma of the fourth ventricle,* showing both characteristic cell patterns. (1) The formation of canals lined by cubical epithelium (near *C*). (2) The perivascular arrangement of spindle-shaped cells—ependymal spongioblasts (below *B* and *D*). One or other of these patterns usually predominates. The blood vessels are thin-walled and numerous.
Hæmalum and Eosin × 75.

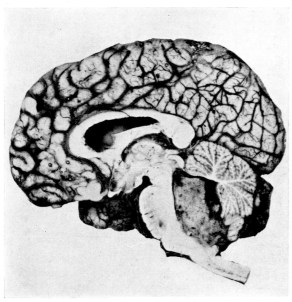

FIG. 210. *Choroidal papilloma of the fourth ventricle* causing obstructive internal hydrocephalus (note the dilated aqueduct and third ventricle).

OLIGODENDROGLIOMA

This is usually a well-demarcated, occasionally cystic, slowly-growing glioma, occurring in the cerebral hemispheres in children and young adults.

The tumour is composed of closely packed sheets of similar cells with a pavemented pattern and (in post-mortem specimens) a characteristic perinuclear halo due to perinuclear cytolysis and cytoplasmic swelling (*see* legend, Fig. 12), which gives a honeycombed or " boxed " appearance to the tumour. Calcification is common. The numerous thin-walled blood vessels have a tendency to branch at obtuse angles, a feature of diagnostic importance (Greenfield).

COLLOID CYST OF THE THIRD VENTRICLE

Occurring only in the third ventricle, where it grows from the anterior wall of the ventricle in a pedunculated form, this rare tumour is thought to arise from the paraphysis (an embryonic outgrowth of the third ventricle).

It reveals itself by intermittent blocking of the foramina of Monro which causes obstructive hydrocephalus. The cyst is filled with gelatinous fluid and has a thin wall formed of connective tissue lined by ciliated columnar epithelium.

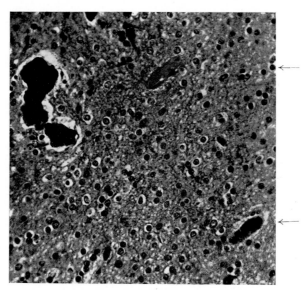

FIG. 211. *Oligodendroglioma.* Biopsy specimen showing the uniform, pavement-like pattern of the cells with round nuclei, the thin-walled blood vessels (arrows) and the calcification (top left) which may show radiographically. In this specimen the cells are more widely spaced than usual and the characteristic " boxing," due to concentric cytoplasmic vacuolation, is not clearly seen.
Hæmalum and Eosin $\times$ 260.

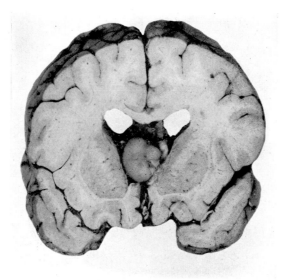

FIG. 212. *Coronal section of brain in the region of the foramen of Monro showing a colloid cyst of the third ventricle* lying in the upper anterior part of the third ventricle.

PINEALOMA

Clinical Note (Fig. 213).—The patient was a man aged 26 years. Since the age of 5 years he had suffered from occasional attacks of frontal headache, lasting never more than a day, first unilateral and then bilateral, accompanied by vomiting. The pupils reacted sluggishly to stimulation, but all eye movements were normal. (It is usual in cases of pinealoma for upward movement of the eyes to be impaired. Paralysis of conjugate upward movement results from pressure of the tumour on the roof or tectum of the midbrain.) X-ray examination showed evidence of long-standing hydrocephalus.

Fig. 213 shows a tumour of 3·5 × 2·5 × 2·5 cm. diameters growing at the site of the pineal and extending mainly forwards into the third ventricle, overhanging the entrance to the cerebral aqueduct and probably producing valvular obstruction. The lateral ventricles and third ventricle are dilated.

Microscopically it showed itself to be a well-differentiated pinealoma, composed of two cell types, one large and epithelioid in appearance, the other small and lymphocytic, thus resembling the pineal of a normal fœtus. Tumours in this region are quite often teratomatous, and Russell (1944) has suggested that such tumours, similar histologically to spheroidal cell carcinoma of the testis, should be considered as atypical teratomata.

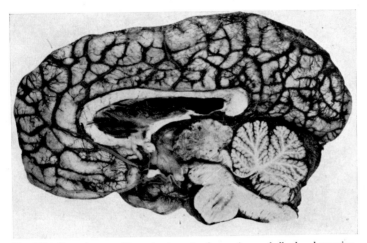

FIG. 213. *Sagittal section of brain showing a pinealoma* acting as a ball valve obstruction at the upper end of the cerebral aqueduct. There is slight involvement of the superior corpora quadrigemina, but the main effect is one of obstructive internal hydrocephalus.

SECONDARY CARCINOMA

Clinical Note (Fig. 214).—The patient, a man of 63 years, had a focal fit on the day prior to admission. *Autopsy* revealed a bronchial carcinoma, with multiple metastases.

Fig. 214 shows some of the many blood-borne metastases to the brain. Note that they are multiple, whereas gliomata are almost invariably solitary. Metastases are often spherical, are sharply demarcated from the surrounding nervous tissue and may show central necrosis, liquefaction or cyst formation. Histologically they resemble the primary tumour. Intracranial metastases, especially from bronchial carcinomata, are quite common.

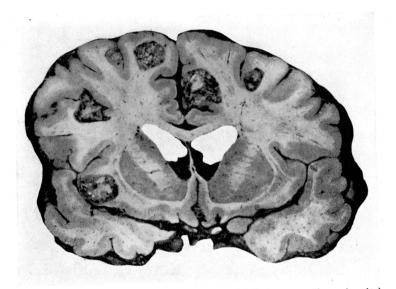

FIG. 214. *Coronal section of brain showing multiple well-defined metastases from a bronchial carcinoma.* The appearances might suggest a glioma, but gliomata almost invariably occur singly, and are not usually so well demarcated from the surrounding brain.

TUMOURS OF THE COVERINGS OF THE NERVOUS SYSTEM

The tumours which arise from the coverings of the nervous system may be divided into :—

(1) Central : *A.* Meningioma (endothelioma) of brain and cord.

                   B. Neurofibroma (neurinoma) (*e.g.*, of acoustic nerve or spinal nerve root).

(2) Peripheral : Neurofibroma (Schwannoma, neurinoma, neurolemmoma).

(3) Central and Peripheral : Neurofibromatosis (von Recklinghausen's disease).

MENINGIOMA

The meningiomata arise from the meninges, usually from the endothelium which lies on the external surface of the arachnoid, and is heaped into focal cellular masses, especially in the arachnoidal villi. Meningiomata may be predominantly fibrous : or predominantly cellular (with cell groups resembling arachnoidal endothelial masses (Fig. 217) and are then often psammomatous (*psammos = sand*) (Fig. 218) ; but they may be predominantly vascular (angioblastic meningioma). They invaginate but do not infiltrate the brain or cord (Figs. 215 and 216). They derive their blood supply from the overlying dura (or from the arachnoid in the uncommon meningioma of the lateral ventricle), not from the brain or cord (Fig. 216).

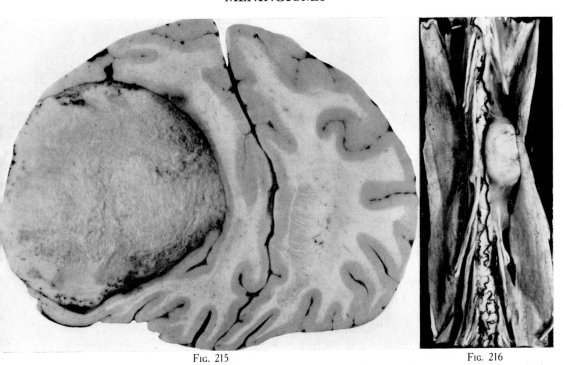

FIG. 215   FIG. 216

FIG. 215.   *Coronal section of brain showing a massive left-sided meningioma.*   Note the granular friable uniform surface and the invagination but not invasion of the cerebral tissue.

FIG. 216.   *Dorsal aspect of thoracic cord showing a right-sided meningioma.*   The main body of the tumour is deep to the arachnoid, which can be seen falling back on to the surface of the cord above and below the tumour.   On the right side the superficial aspect of the tumour is attached to the dura for its blood supply.

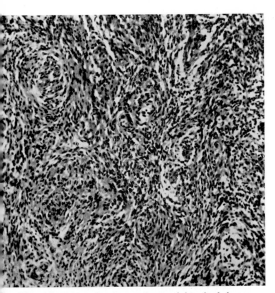

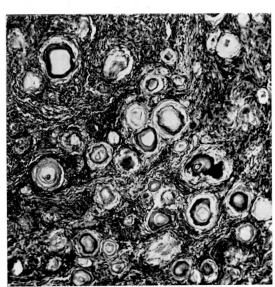

FIG. 217.   *Meningioma* showing a mixture of the whorled pattern typical of arachnoidal endothelial cells and the fasciculated arrangement of elongated bipolar cells (fibroblasts).
Hæmalum and Eosin × 100.

FIG. 218.   *Psammomatous type of meningioma* showing numerous calcified bodies (calcospherites).

Hæmalum and Eosin × 100.

ACOUSTIC NEUROFIBROMA (NEURINOMA)

Fig. 219 is of an acoustic neurofibroma or cerebello-pontine angle tumour on the left side. It has a smooth nodular surface. The 5th nerve appears at the upper pole of the tumour, while the 7th nerve runs over its superior surface. The 8th nerve is incorporated in the tumour and the 9th, 10th and 11th nerves run over its infero-medial surface.

Microscopically (Fig. 220) it is composed of interweaving streams of very elongated bipolar cells with elongated nuclei of varying size. The cells are closely associated with parallel running reticulin fibres. Nuclear pallisading is sometimes present.

Clinically.—Owing to its site and slow-growing nature, focal symptoms precede general symptoms as an almost invariable rule. For long the sole complaints may be of noises in the ear and increasing deafness. Giddy sensations follow as vestibular fibres come under pressure. Headache and early papilloedema, general symptoms of raised intracranial pressure due to obstructive hydrocephalus, appear. As the tumour expands, both sensory 5th (*e.g.*, corneal reflex disappears) and 7th nerves are apt to be damaged. The motor 5th is not involved until later. The 6th rarely suffers. Ipsilateral cerebellar symptoms then occur and the pyramidal tract may be affected, either on the same side of the brain, or on the opposite side by pressure of the opposite pyramid, in the pons, against the petrous bone (after Kinnier Wilson). On lumbar puncture the cerebro-spinal fluid is under increased pressure and the protein content is raised.

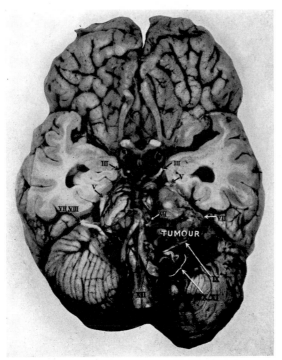

FIG. 219. *Undersurface of brain showing a left-sided acoustic neurofibroma*, growing in the cerebello-pontine angle. The 8th nerve is incorporated in the tumour mass.

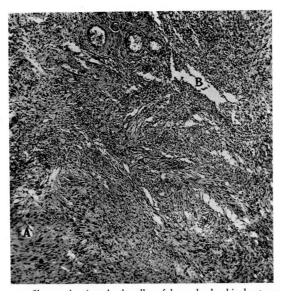

FIG. 220. *Acoustic neurofibroma*, showing the bundles of long slender bipolar tumour cells, sometimes with a suggestion of nuclear palisading (near *A*). On cross section these bundles have a cribriform (many small holes) appearance. Portions of the tumour (above *B*) have a degenerate appearance, the cells being loosely packed and rather stellate (areolar regions). The majority of the blood vessels are well formed (*C*), but large blood-filled spaces with walls formed of tumour cells are also found (not illustrated). The space around the letter *B* is an artefact. *Hæmalum and Eosin* × 45.

163

PERIPHERAL NEUROFIBROMA
(Neurinoma, neurolemmoma, Schwannoma)

Closely akin histologically to the acoustic neurofibroma are the tumours which are sometimes found singly upon the spinal nerve roots or peripheral nerves. They are simple tumours, encapsulated, composed of an over-growth of cells which have some of the characteristics of Schwann cells and some of the characteristics of the fibrous (endoneurial and perineurial) sheaths of the nerves. Because of these features there is debate as to whether they arise primarily from Schwann cells or from the mesodermal elements of the nerves, hence the multiplicity of names for these tumours.

It is thought by some observers that the solitary peripheral neuro-fibromata belong to a different disease process from neurofibromatosis. In support of this it is stated that, in the solitary peripheral neurofibromata, myelinated fibres are found predominantly in the periphery of the tumour (Fig. 222), whilst in neurofibromatosis they run through the substance of the tumour (Figs. 224 and 225). Others however consider that there is no definite histological basis for the separation of these two conditions. Greenfield (1938), with an experience of many cases, proven by autopsy to be neurofibromatosis, has, especially in the nodular form of neurofibromatosis, observed many swellings on the peripheral nerves which were similar histologically to " solitary peripheral neurofibromata." In such nodules, obviously part of neurofibromatosis, the myelinated fibres were found chiefly at the periphery of the tumour. In his opinion there is no essential difference between the structure of the conditions here described as acoustic neurofibroma, solitary peripheral neurofibroma and neurofibromatosis.

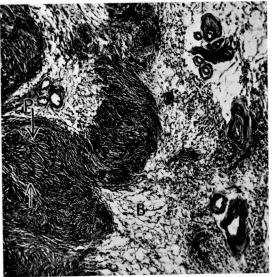

FIG. 221. *Peripheral neurofibroma* showing the two classical regions (Antoni).
(1) Regions of fasciculated elongated cells with pallisaded nuclei (*P*) and
(2) Reticulated (net-like) regions (*B*) with fewer fibres, irregularly vacuolated scattered cells and hyaline fibrous thickening of the vessel walls (*V*).
Hæmalum and Eosin × 70.

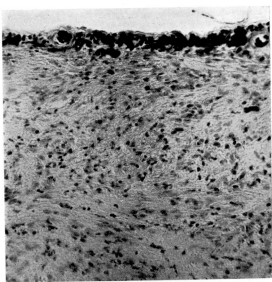

FIG. 222. *Peripheral neurofibroma* stained to show myelin sheaths. Note the myelin sheaths (top of picture) lying at the periphery of the tumour. Compare Figs. 224 and 225.
Spielmeyer's myelin stain × 220.

NEUROFIBROMATOSIS
(VON RECKLINGHAUSEN'S DISEASE)

This is a system disease, of a neoplastic (benign or sometimes malignant) nature, affecting the supporting structure of the nervous system. It may show some or many of the following features :—

(1) Central astrocytoma or ependymoma (not glioblastoma).

(2) Multiple meningiomata.

(3) Fibroblastic swellings upon cranial, spinal and peripheral nerves, upon autonomic nerves and upon nerve endings in the skin. Such swellings may be solitary, or multiple and confluent. The swellings may be firm in consistence and situated principally towards one aspect of the nerve (*nodular type*, Fig. 223); or they may be soft and gelatinous and situated in the long axis of the nerve (*plexiform type*, Fig. 224). They may become sarcomatous.

(4) Pigmented regions in the skin.

(5) Bony changes (softening).

Figs. 223 and 226 show neural and cutaneous nodules. The skin shows café-au-lait pigmentation.

Microscopically.—In the neural swellings of the nodular type the nerve fibres are situated principally towards the periphery of a compact fibrous tissue overgrowth (as in Fig. 222), whilst in the plexiform type of swelling the nerve fibres can be seen passing through the more central part of the rather œdematous fibrous tissue overgrowth of the endo-, peri- or epineurium (Figs. 224 and 225).

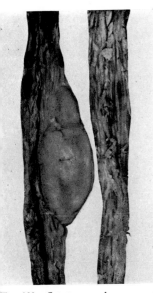

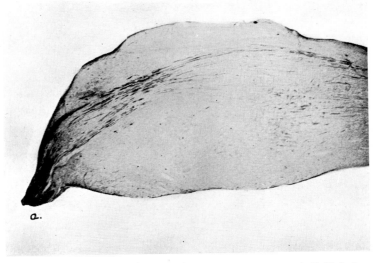

By courtesy of The British Journal of Ophthalmology.

FIG. 223. *Sciatic nerves from a case of neurofibromatosis of nodular type, showing the swelling on the left sciatic nerve.*

FIG. 224. *Longitudinal section of a swelling on a nerve, from a case of neurofibromatosis of plexiform type, showing the nerve entering at (a) and its fibres spreading out within the substance of the swelling. The apparent discontinuity of the fibres is due to the plane of section. Myelin sheath stain × 6.*

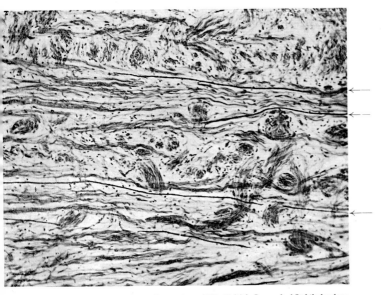

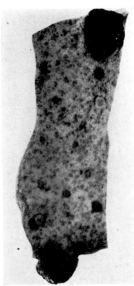

By courtesy of The British Journal of Ophthalmology.

FIG. 225. *Higher power view of a swelling on a nerve in neurofibromatosis of plexiform type, showing the axis cylinders (arrows) passing through the middle of loose connective tissue. Compare Fig. 222. Axis cylinder stain × 110.*

FIG. 226. *Cutaneous nodules, some pedunculated, from a case of neurofibromatosis, showing the often associated café - au - lait pigmentation.*

HÆMANGIOBLASTOMA OF CEREBELLUM

Clinical Note.—The patient was a woman aged 26 years. Three months before death she experienced drooping of the upper eyelids and two months before death suffered from occipital headaches, vomiting, sleepiness and dizziness. Examination revealed marked bilateral papillœdema, a left lower 7th nerve palsy, and dysdiadochokinesis of the left upper limb. X-ray examination of the skull was negative. On lumbar puncture the cerebro-spinal fluid pressure was 490 mm. (of C.S.F.) and the cellular content was 1 cell per c.mm.

Fig. 227 shows the tumour of the left cerebellar hemisphere consisting of a mural nodule and a cyst. The mural nodule consisted *microscopically* (Fig. 228) of innumerable small vascular spaces formed by endothelial cells. Between the blood spaces were aggregations of lipoid-containing endothelial cells. The cyst was produced by transudation of protein-rich fluid, from the blood in the vessels of the mural nodule, and its wall consisted of compressed cerebellar tissue.

This tumour, in this form, is found almost exclusively below the tentorium cerebelli. It is sometimes associated with angiomatosis of the retina (von Hippel's disease), when the combined lesion is known as Lindau's disease, a combination which may be associated with cystic pancreas and cystic kidneys.

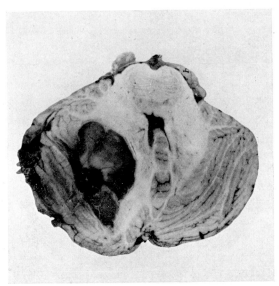

Fig. 227. *Horizontal section of cerebellum containing the dark tumour nodule of a hæmangioblastoma* and the surrounding clear fluid filled cyst, the wall of which is formed of compressed and slightly gliosed cerebellar tissue.

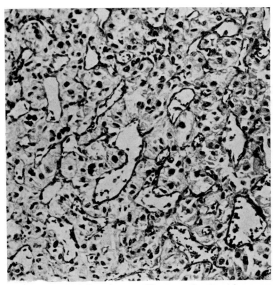

Fig. 228. *Cerebellar hæmangioblastoma* showing the very numerous capillary blood vessels, lined by endothelial cells and separated by vacuolated (lipoid-containing) endothelial cells. *Hæmalum and Eosin* × 150.

PITUITARY ADENOMA

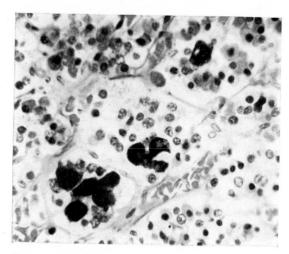

Fig. 229. *Normal human pituitary (pars anterior)* showing the meshwork of thin-walled capillaries to which should be attached the pituitary epithelial cells—the chromophobe (colour fearing) cells with their almost unstained cytoplasm; the chromophile (colour loving) cells with either bluish (basiphilic) or reddish (eosinophilic) granules in the cytoplasm.
Pyrrol blue Eosin × 300.

Tumours of the pituitary almost invariably affect the anterior lobe and are adenomata of either chromophobe or chromophil (eosinophil or basiphil) cells. Chromophobe adenomas are much more common than eosinophil adenomas, mixed adenomas are less common and basiphil adenomas (if allowed as true tumours) are very rare. The pituitary tumours show themselves by their effect upon hormone production and by being space-occupying lesions.

The chromophobe adenoma is composed of cells which have not developed secretory granules. Usually large, this tumour is associated chiefly with hypopituitrism (from pressure on the rest of the gland) and with pressure signs upon the optic chiasm.

The eosinophil adenoma is not usually very large, but it is associated with an over-production of the growth hormone. This will produce gigantism if the epiphyses have not ossified, or acromegaly (enlargement of the acral or peripheral portions of the body such as hands, feet and lower jaw) if the epiphyses have ossified. Sometimes the tumour is formed of cells richly endowed with eosinophilic granules (Fig. 233), sometimes the tumour is larger but the cells have only a scattering of eosinophilic granules at the periphery (transitional or pre-eosinophil adenoma (Fig. 232)).

The basiphil adenoma may be symptomless or may be associated with Cushing's syndrome of obesity, hirsuitism, hypertension, polycythæmia, glycosuria and hypogonadism. Although this syndrome can occur in the absence of basiphil adenoma, Crooke (1935) considers that it is always associated with a hyaline change in the cytoplasm of some of the basiphil cells.

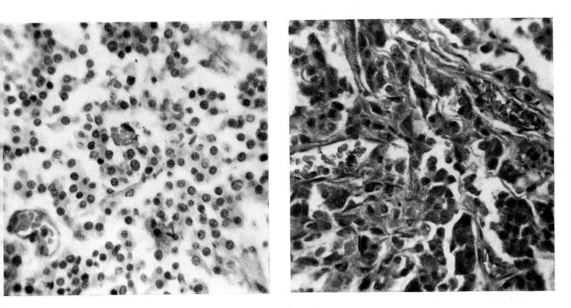

Fig. 230

Fig. 231

Fig. 230. *Chromophobe adenoma of the pars anterior of the pituitary* showing the preservation of the normal vascular pattern, with solid alveolar masses of chromophobe cells, showing regular nuclei, no mitotic figures and only a little faintly staining cytoplasm. (The tumour cells are less closely packed than normal in this biopsy specimen.) *Pyrrol blue Eosin* × 300.

Fig. 231. *Basiphil adenoma of the pars anterior of the pituitary*, from a case without Cushing's syndrome, showing the thin-walled capillaries and the solid alveolar pattern of the tumour cells of similar type with basiphilic cytoplasm. *Pyrrol blue Eosin* × 300.

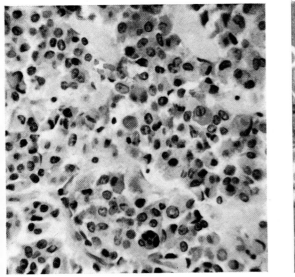

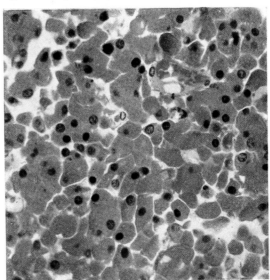

Fig. 232

Fig. 233

Fig. 232. *Pre-eosinophil adenoma of the pars anterior of the pituitary*, from a case of acromegaly, showing (1) the thin-walled capillaries, (2) the loss of normal alveolar pattern, and (3) the tumour cells, some with large nuclei, some binucleated, mostly with much pale staining cytoplasm, some with a dusting of eosinophilic granules at the periphery of the cells and a few with many eosinophilic granules. *Pyrrol blue Eosin* × 300.

Fig. 233. *Eosinophil adenoma of the pars anterior of the pituitary*, from a case of acromegaly, showing the tumour cells with their cytoplasm packed with eosinophilic granules. *Pyrrol blue Eosin* × 300.

CYSTIC EPITHELIAL SUPRAPITUITARY TUMOUR
(CRANIOPHARYNGIOMA)

Fig. 235, of a sagittal section of brain, shows a tumour, lying above the pituitary, which had grown upwards and completely filled the cavity of the third ventricle. The tumour was multicystic, of gritty consistence (opaque particles were visible in an X-ray photograph) and was sharply demarcated from the surrounding brain. Histologically (Fig. 236) such a tumour consists of islands of epithelial cells lying in a stroma containing a mixture of collagen and neuroglia. Calcification may occur in either region. The epithelial islands have an outer layer of columnar cells, like the basal cells of the epidermis, and inside this layer is a mass of squamoid cells, like the squamous cells of the epidermis. Sometimes these islands look like embryonic teeth (adamantinoma). Some of the tumours are predominantly cystic, some are solid. They usually affect children, but may occur in adults.

These tumours arise in this situation as a result of the embryological development of the pituitary (Fig. 234). The pituitary is formed by the fusion of two outgrowths, one from above, a process of the floor of the third ventricle which forms the pars posterior or pars nervosa ; and one from below, an invaginated fold of ectoderm from the roof of the fœtal mouth (Rathke's pouch), which grows up and forms the pars anterior, pars inter-media and pars tuberalis. The cellular connection between the mouth and the pituitary (the hypophyseal duct, craniopharyngeal, or more correctly, craniobuccal canal) atrophies, but epithelial cell residues may remain in the pars tuberalis and from such residues the tumour arises. As it grows it seems to stimulate the glia of the pituitary stalk (infundibulum) so that glial overgrowth takes place and separates the epithelial islands.

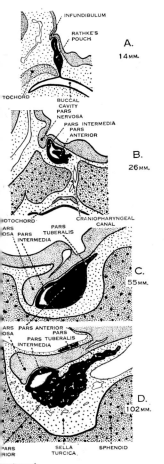

*234. Diagram illustrating the develop-
ment of the pituitary. See text.*

236. Craniopharyngioma showing (1) the islands of
.elial cells (centre), with peripheral columnar cells
ing centrally through squamous cells into spidery cells,
ith cyst formation (top right) ; (2) The collagenous and
overgrowth between the islands (lower left) ; (3) The
ication (top left) which may occur in the epithelial islands
in the overgrowth of collagen and neuroglia, as here.
Hæmalum and Eosin × 75.

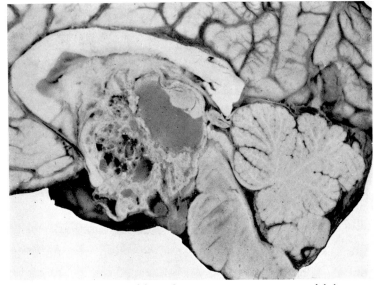

FIG. 235. *Sagittal section of brain showing a cystic suprapituitary epithelial tumour,
invaginating the brain and filling the third ventricle. The large cystic spaces with
colloidal fluid content are clearly seen.*

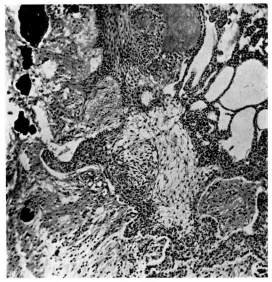

FIG. 236

GANGLIONEUROMA

This tumour of ganglion cells is exceedingly rare in the central nervous system, but it is not uncommon in the peripheral nervous system, in relation to the ganglia of the autonomic nervous system and the adrenal medulla (which are derived from the ectodermal neural crest). It is a slow-growing encapsulated tumour.

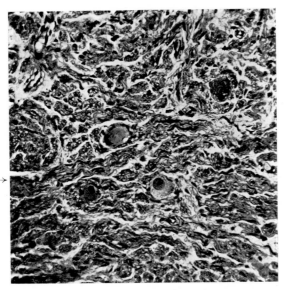

FIG. 237. *Ganglioneuroma*, from the peripheral nervous system, showing a focus of nerve cells (note the large nucleolus). The rest of the tissue consists of Schwann cells and nerve fibres, with a small amount of fine connective tissue, though all these features cannot be clearly seen here. A band of parallel-running Schwann cells can be seen at arrow: these bundles have a fenestrated appearance on cross section.
Hæmalum and Eosin × 200.

SECTION X
ERRORS IN DEVELOPMENT
DEVELOPMENT OF THE NERVOUS SYSTEM

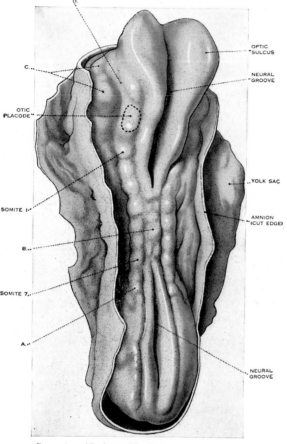

By courtesy of Professors Hamilton, Boyd and Mossman.

FIG. 238. *The dorsal aspect of a reconstruction of a somite human embryo of about the 22nd day. Modified from Payne (1925). The neural groove is being enclosed at (B).*

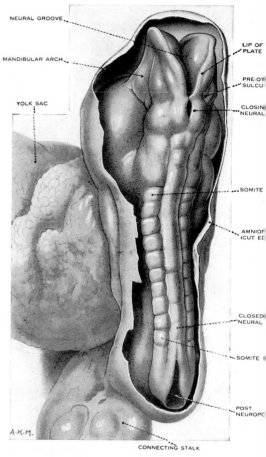

By courtesy of Professors Hamilton, Boyd and Mossman.

FIG. 239. *The dorsal aspect of a reconstruction of a 10 somite human embryo of about the 23rd day. Modified from Corner (1929). The enclosure of the neural groove has spread further.*

The nervous system develops from a specialized strip of surface ectoderm (the neural plate), which becomes grooved (neural groove) and then tubularized (neural tube) and buried below the surface by the upward and medial growth of a mass of mesoderm on either side. It is important to realize that the nervous system does not develop by itself, but is dependent upon the presence, below it, of properly developing mesoderm.

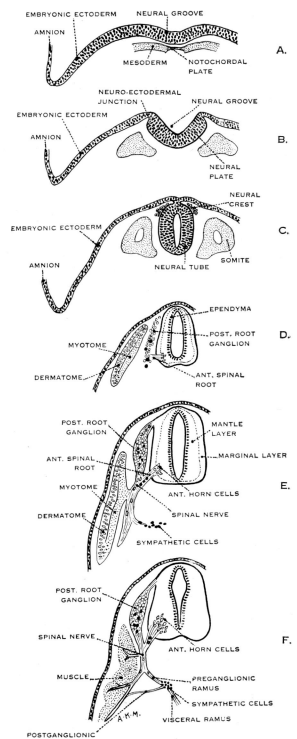

Fig. 240. *Schematic sections through the neural groove, neural tube and their derivatives in successively older (A-F) human embryos. The differentiation of the myotome and dermatome from the somite is also shown.*

By courtesy of Professors
Hamilton, Boyd and Mossman.

RACHISCHIS

(rachis=spine+schisis=cleft)

If the mesodermic growth around the developing nervous system is deficient, then the brain
and cord lie, to a greater or lesser extent, open
upon the surface. In an anencephalic fœtus
(Figs. 243 and 244) the brain and cord lie almost
completely upon the surface (a complete posterior
rachischisis). The least severe form of faulty
closure is spina bifida occulta.

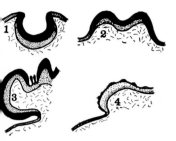

FIG. 241. *Stages in the production of anencephaly.* 1. Non-closure of the neural groove. 2. Extroversion of neural tissue. 3. Further stage of so-called extroversion. 4. Final stage, with degeneration of most of the exposed neural tissue as in Fig. 244.

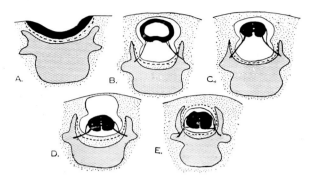

FIG. 242. *Varieties of spina bifida.* *A.* Myelocoele (rachischisis). *B.* Syringomyelocoele. *C.* Meningomyelocoele. *D.* Meningocoele. *E.* Spina bifida occulta. The dura is represented by interrupted lines, the pia-arachnoid by continuous lines.

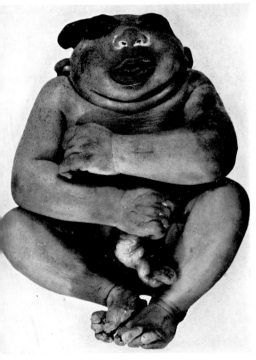

FIG. 243

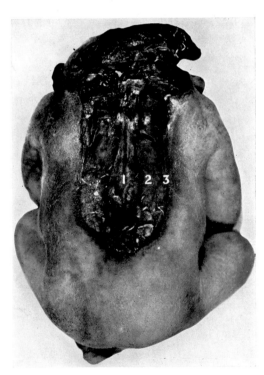

FIG. 244

FIG. 243. *Anencephalic fœtus anterior aspect.* Note the failure of development of the head superior to the eyes.

FIG. 244. *Anencephalic fœtus, dorsal aspect,* showing complete posterior rachischisis. Neither brain nor cord has sunk below the surface owing to the failure of development of the skull and spine. The various zones of the exposed cord region are : 1. Area medullo-vasculosa (flattened rudimentary spinal cord covered with cylindrical epithelium. Such epithelium is the normal covering of a patent neural canal). 2. Area epithelio-serosa (very vascular exposed pia-arachnoid). 3. Zona dermatica (skin).

ARNOLD-CHIARI MALFORMATION AND SYRINGOMYELOCOELE

This condition, described by Arnold (1894) and Chiari (1895) consists of a brainstem and spinal abnormality. Leptomeningeal thickening is present around the rudimentary cerebellum and medulla, which project in a cone-shaped mass through the foramen magnum (Figs. 245 and 246). The upper spinal nerve roots run outwards and upwards instead of at right angles to the cord or slightly downwards (Fig. 246). In the lumbar region a syringomyelocoele is almost invariably present (Figs. 247, 248 and 249). There is an obstructive internal hydrocephalus.

One view of the pathogenesis is as follows. Normally until the third month of foetal life the cord occupies the whole length of the spinal canal. Thereafter the vertebral column grows relatively faster in length, so that, by full term, the cord ends at the third lumbar vertebra. If the cord is anchored at its lower end, by such an abnormality as syringomyelocoele, then traction is exerted in a downward direction. This tends to pull the medulla and cerebellum down through foramen magnum and leads to imperfect development of the cerebellum. By impacting the brainstem and cerebellum in foramen magnum it leads to partial obstruction of the apertures of the fourth ventricle, and thus to obstructive hydrocephalus.

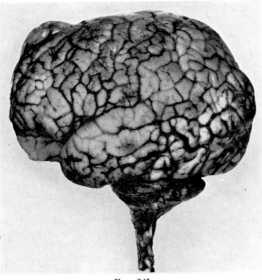

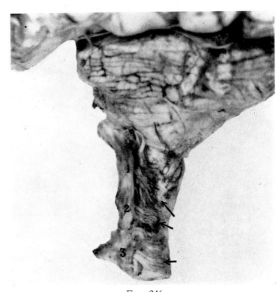

Fig. 245   Fig. 246

Fig. 245. *Arnold-Chiari malformation.* Lateral view of brain showing the rudimentary " turnip-shaped " hindbrain.

Fig. 246. *Arnold-Chiari malformation* showing the rudimentary cerebellum, the thickening of the leptomeninges in the region of foramen magnum (not clearly visible) and the way in which the upper cervical nerve roots, 1, 2, 3, run upwards instead of horizontally.

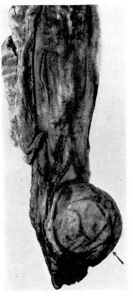

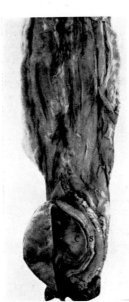

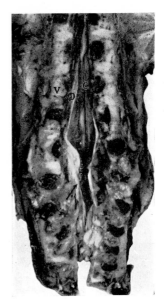

Fig. 247   Fig. 248   Fig. 249

Fig. 247. *Arnold-Chiari malformation.* External view of syringomyelocoele (arrows). The skin and subcutaneous tissues have been removed from the rest of the spinal column.

Fig. 248. *Arnold-Chiari malformation.* The syringomyelocoele has been partially opened showing the cystic cord substance (C) and the cut edge of the skin and subcutaneous tissues (S) of the sac. *See also* Fig. 242 B.

Fig. 249. *Arnold-Chiari malformation.* View of the spinal canal from the anterior aspect. The vertebral bodies (V) have been largely removed. The dura (D) has been opened. The spinal cord (C) disappears below, into the sac of the syringomyelocoele. There it becomes cystic. The lumbo-sacral nerve roots (arrow) emerge again to continue their normal course, functionally useless, for they come from imperfectly developed cord.

181

AGYRIA (LISSENCEPHALY)

(No gyri) *(Smooth brain)*

Clinical Note.—The patient was a male infant aged 1 year 7 months, whose birth was normal. When two weeks old a squint was noticed and fits developed at the age of $5\frac{1}{2}$ months. He was mentally defective and noisy unless under sedatives.

Fig. 250 shows the cerebrum with a lack of the normal gyral pattern, except in the medial occipital and hippocampal regions.

Fig. 251 shows a coronal section of the brain. The basal ganglia are healthy. The thickness of the hemisphere can be divided into four zones :—

(1) A thin and attenuated cortex.

(2) A broad middle zone composed of radial bundles of myelinated fibres between which lie radially elongated masses of grey matter containing many nerve cells of immature appearance.

(3) A smaller but better developed white-matter layer.

(4) Normal ependyma lining the ventricles.

The condition is one of arrested development. The middle zone (2) corresponds to the one which is present at the fourth or fifth month of foetal life when neuroblasts make their way from the ependymal layer to the cortex. It is interesting to note the relative normality of the cerebellum and of the hippocampal and calcarine cortex, all of which are ontogenetically and phylogenetically early developed regions.

MICROGYRIA

(Small gyri)

This is a maldevelopment, which may be due to an error of development or secondary to an inflammatory or destructive process in foetal life. The narrowing of the cortical gyri is often associated with loss of nerve cells and laminar pattern and extensive loss of the underlying white matter. The process may be diffuse or localized (Fig. 252).

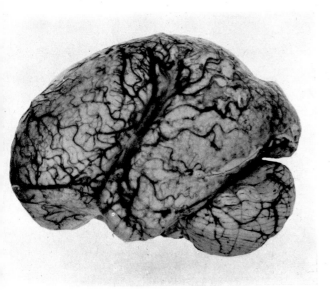

FIG. 250. *Agyria.* Lateral aspect of brain, showing the lack of cerebral gyri. They have developed normally in the cerebellum.

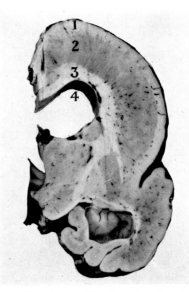

FIG. 251. *Agyria.* Coronal section of cerebral hemisphere at midbrain level, showing the lack of gyri except in the hippocampal region. The various layers of the cerebral tissue are described in the text.

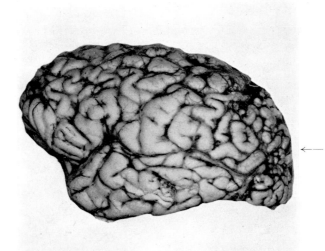

FIG. 252. *Microgyria.* View of lateral aspect of left cerebral hemisphere. The arrow points to the occipital microgyria.

TUBEROUS SCLEROSIS

Tuberous sclerosis is characterized by the presence of large firm glial nodules (said to be of the consistence and appearance of a tuber such as a raw potato), in the cerebral cortex (Figs. 253, 254A and 256), and nodules of glial overgrowth projecting into the ventricles (Figs. 254B and 255). Sometimes these nodules become neoplastic, forming tumours, some of which are spongioblastomata (Fig. 254C).

It is usually associated with adenoma sebaceum of the skin of the face (Fig. 257) (which does not generally become noticeable until the age of puberty) and with congenital abnormalities, such as rhabdomyomata (tumours of striped muscle) of the heart (Fig. 258) and multiple embryonic tumours of the kidneys.

In the cortical nodules the laminar pattern is grossly distorted, the subpial astrocytic layer shows a dense overgrowth and there are foci of giant astrocytes (Fig. 256) and giant nerve cells.

The *pathogenesis* of the condition is obscure. It is a developmental anomaly probably both dysplastic (misformation) and neoplastic (new growth). Neoplasia probably develops in tissues which have developed abnormally from their mother cells. Not only ectoderm is involved, for there are congenital abnormalities of mesoderm as well. Similar combined ectodermal and mesodermal abnormalities may be found in neurofibromatosis.

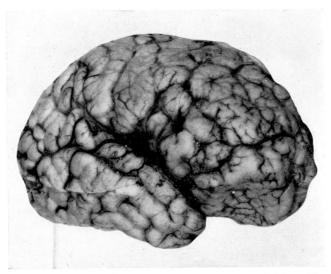

FIG. 253. *Tuberous sclerosis.* Brain from a five weeks old baby. The regions of cortical hardness are very difficult to see, very easy to appreciate by palpation.

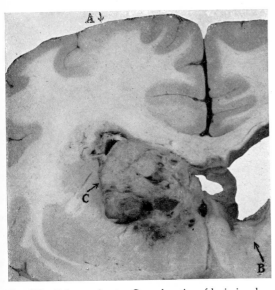

FIG. 254. *Tuberous sclerosis.* Coronal section of brain in a boy of sixteen years, showing (*A*) region of cortical hardness, (*B*) nodule of glial overgrowth projecting into the lateral ventricle, (*C*) spongioblastic tumour which has developed from one of the ventricular nodules.

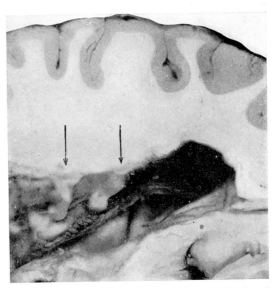

FIG. 255. *Tuberous sclerosis.* Horizontal section of right lateral ventricle in the same patient as Fig. 254. The arrows point to nodules of glial overgrowth projecting into the ventricle. The choroid plexus can be seen running along the floor of the ventricle.

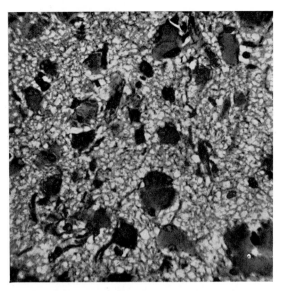

FIG. 256. *Tuberous sclerosis.* Focus of giant cells in a cortical nodule. Some have two nuclei. All those shown here are giant astrocytes, but giant nerve cells are also found.
Hæmalum and Eosin × 350.

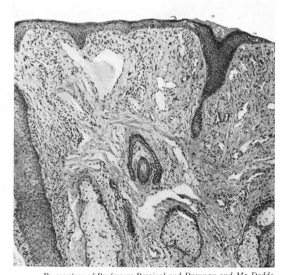

By courtesy of Professors Percival and Drennan and Mr Dodds.

FIG. 257. *Adenoma sebaceum*, showing the numerous blood spaces of varying sizes. This malformation is a combination of angiomatous tissue and sebaceous glandular hyperplasia.
Hæmalum and Eosin × 70.

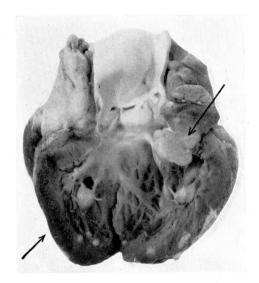

FIG. 258. *Tuberous sclerosis.* Heart from the same patient as Fig. 253. The arrows point to some of the rhabdomyomata. The head of the upper arrow lies upon the cut surface of a large tumour.

CAPILLARY TELANGIECTASIS

(telos=end+aggeion=vessel+ektasis=dilatation)

The normal vascular system may be considered as developing from a primitive capillary network. Sometimes the capillary network is not properly remoulded and a capillary telangiectasis results; sometimes the venular side of the developing vascular system shows malformation and a venous angioma results: sometimes the capillary network is over-absorbed and the blood from the arteries passes directly into the veins (arterio-venous fistula or aneurysm). All these conditions can be accounted for as developmental anomalies, dysplasias *(dus=ill+plassein=to form)* or hamartomata *(hamartia=error)* of blood vessels, distinct from the neoplasia (new formation) which results in the hæmangioblastoma of the cerebellum.

The microscopical pictures (Figs. 259 and 260) are of a clinically silent telangiectasis, which appeared macroscopically as a sort of " peppered " appearance in the white matter of the cerebrum. The telangiectasis was drained by one large venous channel.

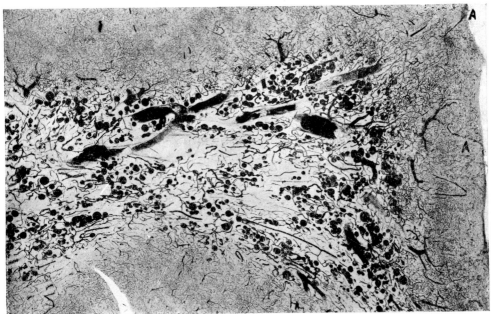

By courtesy of The Journal of Pathology and Bacteriology.

FIG. 259. *Capillary telangiectasis. General vascular pattern.* The main body of the abnormality lies in the white matter, surrounded by cortex. At (*A*) there are communications with cortical arterioles, whilst the large radicles of the draining venous channel can be seen deeper in. *Thick frozen section, 200μ thick, stained by Pickworth's benzidine method which stains the blood corpuscles and thereby demonstrates the vascular pattern* × 8.

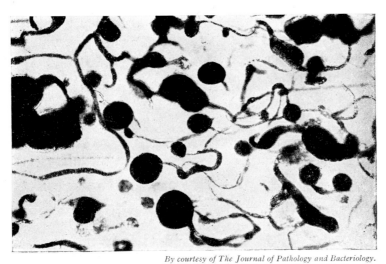

By courtesy of The Journal of Pathology and Bacteriology.

FIG. 260. *Capillary telangiectasis. Higher power view of portion of Fig.* 259, showing fusiform and saccular dilatations of capillary channels × 55.

VENOUS ANGIOMA

A congenital abnormality of the vascular tree which may be any size from a small varix to serpentine masses of enormously dilated veins. It may lie superficially in the leptomeninges or at any depth in the brain.

ARTERIOVENOUS ANGIOMA

A congenital abnormality of the vascular tree with both an arterial and a venous component. The *illustration* (Fig. 262) is of a portion of the brain of a man, aged 66 years, who was admitted to hospital in an unconscious state and died six days later from respiratory infection. Five years before admission he had a subarachnoid hæmorrhage from which he recovered, but was left with dizziness of increasing severity.

At autopsy the brain was swollen and there was enlargement of the veins over the left cerebral hemisphere. A coronal section of the left hemisphere showed that the temporal lobe was occupied by a collection of relatively thin-walled vascular channels, varying in size up to 16 mm. diameter. Rupture had occurred at one point and the blood had ploughed its way up into the cerebral substance, simulating clinically a massive cerebral hæmorrhage.

Microscopically the vascular channels within the brain were both arterial and venous. The arterial ones, diagnosed by the presence of an internal elastic lamina, were much more numerous. Their walls frequently showed evidence of degeneration in the form of intimal and subintimal fibrosis, hyaline change and cholesterol deposits. In the media the muscle was poorly developed. In many channels there was both old and new ante-mortem clot.

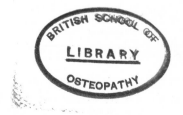

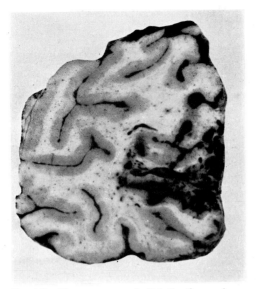

FIG. 261. *Venous angioma.* A clinically silent angioma, in the occipital lobe of a man who died from general paralysis of the insane. Large venous channels can be seen both on the surface and in the depths of the brain.

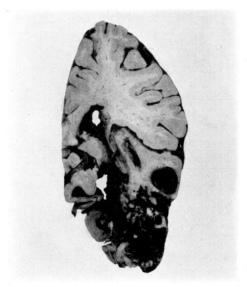

FIG. 262. *Arteriovenous angioma.* Coronal section of left hemisphere at the level of the pineal. The angioma is in the temporal lobe. See text.

REFERENCES

ARNOLD, J. (1894), Myelocyste, Transposition von Gewebskeimen und Sympodie, *Beitr. path. Anat.*, **16**, 1.

BAILEY, P. and CUSHING, H. (1926), Tumours of the Glioma Group, Philadelphia.

BATTEN, F. E. (1903), Three cases of myopathy, infantile type, *Brain*, **26**, 147.

BOLLINGER, O. (1891), Internat. Beitr. z. Wiss. Med. Fest. Rud. Virchow, Berlin.

CAIRNS, H. (1946), Crash helmets, *Brit. Med. J.*, **2**, 322.

CAJAL, S. R. (1909), Histologie du Système Nerveux de l'homme et des vertébrés, Paris, Vol. **1**, p. 508.

CAMPBELL, A. C. P. and BIGGART, J. H. (1939), Wernicke's Encephalopathy (polioencephalitis hæmorrhagica superior) : its alcoholic and non-alcoholic incidence, *J. Path. Bact.*, **48**, 245.

CHIARI, H. (1895), Ueber Veränderungen des Kleinhirns, des Pons und der Medulla oblongata in folge von congenitaler Hydrocephalie des Grosshirns, *Denkschr. Akad. Wiss. Wien*, **63**, 71.

CORNER, G. W. (1929), A well preserved human embryo of 10 somites, *Contr. Embryol. Carneg. Instn.*, **20**, 81.

CROOKE, A. C. (1935), A change in the basophil cells of the pituitary gland common to conditions which exhibit the syndrome attributed to basophil adenoma, *J. Path. Bact.*, **41**, 339.

CUSHING, H. (1932), Intracranial Tumours : Notes upon a series of two thousand verified cases with surgical-mortality percentages pertaining thereto, Springfield, Ill.

DANDY, W. E. (1944), Intracranial arterial aneurysms, Ithaca, New York.

DOTT, N. M. (1944), in Surgery of Modern Warfare, ed. Hamilton Bailey, 3rd edn., Edinburgh, p. 720.

DRENNAN, A. M. (1921), Aneurysms of the larger cerebral arteries, Wellington, New Zealand.

EVANS, W. (1931), The pathology and ætiology of brain abscess, *Lancet*, **1**, 1231 and 1289.

FORBUS, W. P. (1930), On the origin of miliary aneurysms of the superficial arteries, *Bull. Johns Hopkins Hosp.*, **47**, 239.

GLOBUS, J. H. and STRAUSS, I. (1927), Massive cerebral hæmorrhage, *Arch. Neurol. Psychiat., Chicago*, **18**, 215.

GREENFIELD, J. G. (1929), The pathology of measles encephalitis, *Brain*, **52**, 171.

GREENFIELD, J. G. and ELKINGTON, J. ST. C. (1938), Neurofibromatosis, *The British Encyclopaedia of Medical Practice, London*, **9**, 214.

GRINKER, R. R. (1943), Neurology, 3rd edn., Springfield, Ill.

GUTMANN, E. and YOUNG, J. Z. (1944), The re-innervation of muscle after various periods of atrophy, *J. Anat., Lond.*, **78**, 15.

HOFFMANN, J. (1893), Ueber chronische spinale Muskelatrophie im Kindesalter, auf familiärer Basis, *Dtsch. Z. Nervenheilk*, **3**, 427.

HOLBOURN, A. H. S. (1943), Mechanics of head injury, *Lancet*, **2**, 438.

HURST, E. W. (1941), Demyelination : a clinico-pathological and experimental study, *Med. J. Aust.*, **2**, 661.

OPPENHEIM, H. (1900), Ueber allgemeine und localisierte Atonie der Muskulatur (Myatonie) im frühen Kindesalter, *Mschr. Psychiat. Neurol.*, **8**, 232.

PAYNE, F. (1924), General description of a 7-somite embryo, *Contr. Embryol. Carneg. Instn.*, **16**, 117.

PUTNAM, T. J. and ALEXANDER, L. (1939), Disseminated encephalomyelitis : histologic syndrome associated with thrombosis of small cerebral vessels, *Arch. Neurol. Psychiat., Chicago*, **41**, 1087.

RICH, A. R. and MCCORDOCK, H. A. (1933), The pathogenesis of tuberculous meningitis, *Bull. Johns Hopkins Hosp.*, **52**, 5.

RUSSELL, D. S. (1937), Changes in central nervous system following arsphenamine medication, *J. Path. Bact.*, **45**, 357.

RUSSELL, D. S. (1944), The pinealoma : its relationship to teratoma, *J. Path. Bact.*, **56**, 145.

RUSSELL, D. S. (1946), Myocarditis in Friedreich's ataxia, *J. Path. Bact.*, **58**, 739.

DE WARDENER, H. E. and LENNOX, B. (1947), Cerebral beriberi (Wernicke's encephalopathy), *Lancet*, **1**, 11.

WERDNIG, G. (1891), Zwei frühinfantile hereditäre Fälle von progressiver Muskelatrophie unter dem Bilde der Dystrophie, aber auf Neurotischer Basis, *Arch. Psychiat. Nervenkr.*, **22**, 437.

WILSON, S. A. K. (1940), Neurology, London.

WORTIS, H., BUEDING, E., STEIN, M. H. and JOLLIFFE, N. (1942), Pyruvic acid studies in the Wernicke syndrome, *Arch. Neurol. Psychiat., Chicago*, **47**, 215.

YOUNG, J. Z. (1942), The functional repair of nervous tissue, *Physiol. Rev.*, **22**, 318.

YOUNG, J. Z. (1945), Structure, degeneration and repair of nerve fibres, *Nature, Lond.*, **156**, 132

INDEX

Roman type is used for text page number and **bold** *type for illustration figure number*

INDEX

Roman type is used for text page number and **bold** *type for illustration figure number*

INDEX

Roman type is used for text page number and **bold** *type for illustration figure number*

Roman type is used for text page number and **bold** *type for illustration figure number*